Neurology of Pregnancy

Editor

MARY ANGELA O'NEAL

NEUROLOGIC CLINICS

www.neurologic.theclinics.com

Consulting Editor
RANDOLPH W. EVANS

February 2019 • Volume 37 • Number 1

ELSEVIER

1600 John F. Kennedy Boulevard • Suite 1800 • Philadelphia, Pennsylvania, 19103-2899

http://www.theclinics.com

NEUROLOGIC CLINICS Volume 37, Number 1
February 2019 ISSN 0733-8619, ISBN-13: 978-0-323-65475-3

Editor: Stacy Eastman
Developmental Editor: Donald Mumford

Neurologic Clinics (ISSN 0733-8619) is published quarterly by Elsevier Inc., 360 Park Avenue South, New York, NY 10010–1710. Months of issue are February, May, August, and November. Periodicals postage paid at New York, NY, and additional mailing offices. Subscription prices are $323.00 per year for US individuals, $663.00 per year for US institutions, $100.00 per year for US students, $408.00 per year for Canadian individuals, $803.00 per year for Canadian institutions, $427.00 per year for international individuals, $803.00 per year for international institutions, and $210.00 for Canadian and foreign students/residents. To receive student/resident rate, orders must be accompanied by name of affiliated institution, date of term, and the *signature* of program/residency coordinator on institution letterhead. Orders will be billed at individual rate until proof of status is received. Foreign air speed delivery is included in all *Clinics* subscription prices. All prices are subject to change without notice. **POSTMASTER:** Send address changes to *Neurologic Clinics*, Elsevier Health Sciences Division, Subscription Customer Service, 3251 Riverport Lane, Maryland Heights, MO 63043. **Customer Service: Telephone: 1-800-654-2452 (U.S. and Canada); 314-447-8871 (outside U.S. and Canada). Fax: 314-447-8029. E-mail: journalscustomerservice-usa@elsevier.com (for print support); journalsonlinesupport-usa@elsevier.com (for online support).**

Reprints. For copies of 100 or more of articles in this publication, please contact the Commercial Reprints Department, Elsevier Inc., 360 Park Avenue South, New York, New York, 10010-1710; Tel.: +1-212-633-3874; Fax: +1-212-633-3820, and E-mail: reprints@elsevier.com.

Neurologic Clinics is also published in Spanish by Nueva Editorial Interamericana S.A., Mexico City, Mexico.

Neurologic Clinics is covered in *Current Contents/Clinical Medicine, MEDLINE/PubMed (Index Medicus), EMBASE/Excerpta Medica, and PsycINFO, and ISI/BIOMED.*

Contributors

CONSULTING EDITOR

RANDOLPH W. EVANS, MD
Clinical Professor, Department of Neurology, Baylor College of Medicine, Houston, Texas

EDITOR

MARY ANGELA O'NEAL, MD
Director of the Women's Neurology Program, Clinical Director of the Neuroscience Center, Department of Neurology, Brigham and Women's Hospital, Harvard Medical School, Boston, Massachusetts

AUTHORS

SHAMIK BHATTACHARYYA, MD, MS
Assistant Professor, Department of Neurology, Brigham and Women's Hospital, Harvard Medical School, Boston, Massachusetts

REBECCA BURCH, MD
Assistant Professor, Department of Neurology, Staff Physician, John R. Graham Headache Center, Brigham and Women's Hospital, Harvard Medical School, Boston, Massachusetts

ERICA C. CAMARGO, MD, MMSc, PhD
Associate Inpatient Medical Director, Instructor, Department of Neurology, Massachusetts General Hospital, Harvard Medical School, Boston, Massachusetts

STEVEN K. FESKE, MD
Director, Stroke Division, Associate Professor, Department of Neurology, Brigham and Women's Hospital, Harvard Medical School, Boston, Massachusetts

AUBREY L. GILBERT, MD, PhD
Department of Ophthalmology, The Permanente Medical Group, Vallejo, California

CYNTHIA HARDEN, MD
Attending Physician, The Head of the Therapeutic Area of Epilepsy for Xenon Pharmaceuticals, Inc, New York, New York

LIANGGE HSU, MD
Assistant Professor, Department of Radiology, Brigham and Women's Hospital, Boston, Massachusetts

TAMARA B. KAPLAN, MD
Department of Neurology, Neurologist, Partners Multiple Sclerosis Center, Brigham and Women's Hospital, Instructor, Harvard Medical School, Boston, Massachusetts

CHRISTINE LU, MD
Resident Physician, Department of Neurology, Mount Sinai Downtown, New York, New York

ROBERT M. MALLERY, MD
Instructor, Department of Neurology, Harvard Medical School, Brigham and Women's Hospital, Department of Ophthalmology, Massachusetts Eye and Ear, Boston, Massachusetts

MARY ANGELA O'NEAL, MD
Director of the Women's Neurology Program, Clinical Director of the Neuroscience Center, Department of Neurology, Brigham and Women's Hospital, Harvard Medical School, Boston, Massachusetts

SASHANK PRASAD, MD
Associate Professor, Department of Neurology, Harvard Medical School, Brigham and Women's Hospital, Boston, Massachusetts

SOPHIA L. RYAN, MD
Clinical Fellow, Department of Neurology, Brigham and Women's Hospital, Department of Neurology, Massachusetts General Hospital, Harvard Medical School, Boston, Massachusetts

ANEESH B. SINGHAL, MD
Vice Chair, Quality and Safety, Associate Professor, Department of Neurology, Massachusetts General Hospital, Harvard Medical School, Boston, Massachusetts

LAURA STERNICK, MD
Department of Radiology, Brigham and Women's Hospital, Boston, Massachusetts

JANET WATERS, MD, MBA
Division Chief, Women's Neurology, Associate Professor, University of Pittsburgh Medical Center, Pittsburgh, Pennsylvania

WHITNEY W. WOODMANSEE, MD
Professor of Medicine, Director, Neuroendocrine/Pituitary Program, Division of Endocrinology, Diabetes and Metabolism, University of Florida, Gainesville, Florida

Contents

> Pregnancy is a complex physiologic state with hormonal, hemodynamic, hematologic, and immunologic changes at both global and cellular levels affecting brain, heart, pituitary, thyroid, and kidney. There are many situations in which imaging can aid in diagnosis and subsequent treatment of neurologic conditions during pregnancy.

> Multiple sclerosis (MS) and neuromyelitis optica (NMO) are chronic inflammatory demyelinating disorders of the central nervous system that often affect women during childbearing years. Therefore, issues of conception, pregnancy, and delivery are of significant importance to patients and treating physicians. The current review provides updated information regarding the effects of pregnancy on MS and NMO, as well as the available safety data on immunomodulatory MS therapies for pregnant and lactating women. Management issues of women with MS and NMO during conception, gestation, and the postpartum period also are addressed.

> Migraine is the most common cause of headache during pregnancy. Pregnancy increases risk for many causes of headache, including pathologic vascular processes. Headache associated with neurologic signs or symptoms or that is progressive and refractory to treatment; acute in onset; and severe, postural, or different from typical headaches should be evaluated. Work-up should include cerebral and cerebrovascular imaging and monitoring for hypertension. Acetaminophen is first-line symptomatic treatment during pregnancy, and evidence supports triptans rather than butalbital combination analgesics as second-line treatment. Propranolol is preferred preventive treatment, and amitriptyline and verapamil may be considered. Treatment of migraine during lactation is less restrictive than during pregnancy.

> Epilepsy is a prevalent, chronic, and serious neurologic disease affecting many women of childbearing age. Specific concerns, including contraception, fertility, teratogenic risk of antiepileptic drugs, delivery, and

breastfeeding, are addressed in this article. Evidence-based counseling and management strategies are provided to help clinicians and women with epilepsy through the different stages of pregnancy.

Whitney W. Woodmansee

Pregnancy is associated with pituitary enlargement and alterations in hormonal function. Diagnosis of pituitary dysfunction can be challenging during pregnancy due to known changes in hormonal status. Pituitary disorders, particularly adenomas, are relatively common and with medical advancements, more women with pituitary disorders are becoming pregnant. Management includes optimization of hormonal function and close monitoring for signs of tumor progression during pregnancy. Tumor directed medical therapy is generally discontinued during pregnancy but can be re-initiated if there is evidence of tumor growth. Most women do not show aggressive tumor growth during pregnancy and can be successfully managed conservatively until delivery.

Aubrey L. Gilbert, Sashank Prasad, and Robert M. Mallery

The physiologic changes that accompany pregnancy can have important implications for neuro-ophthalmic disease. This article discusses pregnancy-related considerations for meningioma, pituitary disorders, demyelinating disease, myasthenia gravis, thyroid eye disease, idiopathic intracranial hypertension, cerebral venous sinus thrombosis, stroke, migraine, and cranial neuropathies. The article also details the potential neuro-ophthalmic complications of preeclampsia and eclampsia and reviews the use of common diagnostic studies during pregnancy.

Mary Angela O'Neal

This article reviews the common lower extremity postpartum neuropathies, including their incidence, risk factors, clinical features, and treatment. In addition, the rarer complications from neuraxial anesthesia are also discussed.

Janet Waters

Myasthenia gravis is an autoimmune disorder characterized by fluctuating weakness of extraocular and proximal limb muscles. It occurs in 1 in 5000 in the overall population and is 2 times more common in women than men. The onset in women is most common in the third decade, and risk of severe exacerbation occurs most frequently in the year after presentation. The disease does not have an impact on fertility and overlap with pregnancy is expected. This article provides a description of the disease process and its impact on the expecting mother, fetus, and newborn. Management options in pregnancy and lactation are discussed.

Connective tissue disorders are now understood to include autoimmune and genetic diseases affecting organs, blood vessels, and surrounding fascia. Many of these diseases predominantly affect women in child-bearing years and are associated with neurologic complications. Pregnancy can affect disease activity (such as flares of systemic lupus erythematosus), and the diseases can affect pregnancy outcome (such as increased risk of preterm labor). We review the neurologic complications and changes with pregnancy for systemic lupus erythematosus, Sjögren syndrome, idiopathic inflammatory myopathy, and Marfan syndrome.

Pregnancy confers a substantially increased risk of stroke in women. The period of highest risk of stroke is the peripartum/postpartum phase, coinciding with the highest risk for hypertensive disorders of pregnancy and peak gestational hypercoagulability. Hemorrhagic stroke is the most common type of obstetric stroke. Hypertensive disorders of pregnancy are important contributors to obstetric stroke and predispose women to premature cardiovascular disease. The rate of stroke associated with hypertensive disorders of pregnancy has increased in the United States. Other conditions associated with obstetric stroke include posterior reversible encephalopathy, reversible cerebral vasoconstriction syndrome, and cerebral venous sinus thrombosis.

NEUROLOGIC CLINICS

RELATED SERIES

Neuroimaging Clinics
Psychiatric Clinics
Child and Adolescent Psychiatric Clinics

THE CLINICS ARE AVAILABLE ONLINE!
Access your subscription at:
www.theclinics.com

Preface

Introduction to Neurology of Pregnancy

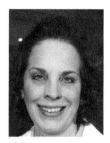

Mary Angela O'Neal, MD
Editor

This issue of *Neurologic Clinics* is devoted to how neurologic conditions may be affected or caused by pregnancy. The normal physiologic changes that occur in pregnancy and postpartum in some instances can predispose to neurologic disease. In addition, pregnancy may affect neurologic disorders as well as the converse: neurologic disorders can affect pregnancy outcomes.

The most common and challenging pregnancy concerns faced by our female patients are addressed. These include neuro-ophthalmologic disorders, management of demyelinating disorders, postpartum neuropathies, management of myasthenia gravis, headache in pregnancy and postpartum, epilepsy, pituitary disorders, stroke, imaging considerations, and connective tissue disorders. Authors were chosen for their known expertise in their subspecialty area.

This issue of *Neurologic Clinics* is meant to be a practical review of disorders and concerns facing treating clinicians in caring for women in their reproductive years. Such concerns include careful planning prior to pregnancy along with attention to potential complications that can occur during pregnancy and in the postpartum period. I

Neurol Clin 37 (2019) ix–x
https://doi.org/10.1016/j.ncl.2018.10.001
0733-8619/19/© 2018 Published by Elsevier Inc.

hope you enjoy reading this issue and learn as much as I did from my expert colleagues.

Mary Angela O'Neal, MD
Department of Neurology
Hale Building of Transformative Medicine
Brigham and Women's Hospital
Harvard Medical School
60 Fenwood Road
Boston, MA 02115, USA

E-mail address:
maoneal@bwh.harvard.edu

Imaging Considerations in Pregnancy

Laura Sternick, MD, Liangge Hsu, MD*

KEYWORDS

- Pregnancy • Radiation safety • Imaging • Stroke • Eclampsia • PRES • RCVS

KEY POINTS

- Overall, diagnostic examinations are safe to perform during pregnancy.
- Deterministic effects are negligible at any gestational age for low-risk examinations. Risks and benefits for noncontrast MR are essentially the same as without pregnancy.
- Computed tomography contrast is safe to use with MR contrast only if necessary.
- There is no need to stop breastfeeding, except when nuclear medicine agents are used.

INTRODUCTION

Pregnancy is a complex interplay of multiple physiologic states maintaining balance between the needs of mother and fetus. This is reflected in hormonal, hemodynamic, hematologic, and immunologic changes at both global and cellular levels. A decrease in brain size and increase in heart, pituitary, thyroid, and kidney sizes secondary to hormonal influences have been observed during pregnancy.[1,2] Circulating hormones also have trophic effect on preexisting neoplasms, such as meningioma, pituitary adenomas, and breast carcinoma.[3] The increased blood volume and clotting factor alterations increase the risk of stroke, especially during the peripartum and postpartum period.[4,5] Hemodynamic and hormonal effects on vessel wall integrity can lead to worsening of aneurysm with possible hemorrhage, whereas prolonged labor may increase risk of infarct from venous thrombosis or dissection.[6,7] In contrast, increased cortisol levels have shown to improve autoimmune diseases such as multiple sclerosis by exerting inhibitory effect on T-cell function[8–10]

With all these pregnancy-related issues, there are many circumstances in which imaging can aid in diagnosis and treatment. Common causes for imaging include stroke, hemorrhage, vascular thrombosis, eclampsia, pituitary issues, and back pain. With potential exposure to radiation and contrast material, it is often required to weigh

Disclosure: Authors have no disclosures to declare.
Department of Radiology, Brigham and Women's Hospital, 75 Francis Street, Boston, MA 02115, USA
* Corresponding author.
E-mail address: LHSU1@bwh.harvard.edu

and balance risks versus benefits. Many helpful guidelines have been established by different groups, including American College of Radiology (ACR), Centers for Disease Control and Prevention, American College of Obstetricians and Gynecologists, and European Society of Urogenital Radiology. There are, however, situations in which the decision-making falls primarily on the physician and patient on a case-by-case basis, emphasizing the importance of understanding the real and not perceived risks of medical imaging.

Radiation comprises both natural (cosmic rays, radon) and manmade sources, including medical (diagnostic and therapeutic) and nonmedical (nuclear fuel and weaponry) uses. In general, emitted radiation is measured in Curies or Becquerels, energy absorbed by mass in rad or gray and relative biological damage in humans in rem or Sievert. X-rays and gamma rays are overall less damaging than neutrons or alpha particles. For x-rays and gamma rays, 1 rad essentially equals equivalent and effective dose (via radiation and tissue weighting factor) of 1 rem/10 millisievert (mSv) all derived from joules/kg.[11] To give some perspective, background radiation is approximately 2.4 mSv per year, a flight from New York to Los Angeles is approximately 5 microsievert/h (about same as 8 dental x-rays), and the legal annual exposure for a nuclear worker is 50 mSv.[12–14] Doses that are greater than 500 mSv will produce some symptoms of radiation poisoning, whereas greater than 6000 mSv can be fatal.[15] Exposure to a single dose all at once causes more damage than an equivalent dose distributed over time.

Much of the radiation effects data came from animal experiments, pregnant patients undergoing therapeutic radiation, and survivors of Hiroshima and Nagasaki.[16–19] It should be noted that these are much higher doses than those encountered in current medical imaging. The risks to the fetus are determined by the gestational age of exposure, and total and rate of dose delivered, which reflects differences in imaging modality and fetus anatomic location.[20–22] Radiation effects are classified into 2 categories: stochastic/random effects versus deterministic/nonrandom effects. Stochastic effects are caused by mutagenesis and carcinogenesis from any dose of radiation and without an exposure threshold. Deterministic effects are dose-related, increase in severity with increased dose, and have an exposure threshold ranging from 50 to 150 mSv.[23] Potential clinical stochastic radiation effects are unrepaired or misrepaired DNA damage leading to cancer, such as leukemia. The dose-dependent risk of leukemia has been estimated at approximately 6% per 1000 mSv exposure in utero.[24] Clinical deterministic effects resulting in cell death can be lethal (spontaneous abortion) or cause central nervous system (CNS) abnormality, cataracts, malformations (100–200 mSv), and growth and mental retardation.

Within the first 2 weeks of gestation, the effect is all or nothing (ie, spontaneous abortion or no effect) for doses greater than 100 mSv. From 3 to 8 weeks during organogenesis, animal studies show growth retardation and malformation at doses greater than 100 to 200 mSv, whereas from 8 to 25 weeks, mental retardation is likely with greater than 500 mSv. From 25 weeks until birth, it is stochastic risk of potential induced neoplasms. At less than 50 mSv, there are no deterministic effects at all stages and from 16 weeks to birth, doses less than 500 mSv are unlikely to cause any deterministic effects, with threshold for congenital effect at approximately 500 to 700 mSv[25] (**Table 1**).

From the imaging standpoint, the effective dose is approximated by the mean skin exposure/film to estimate dose at a certain depth, with measurement affected by patient anatomy, uterus position, and degree of bladder extension.[26] Fetal doses are almost always less than 100 mSv. There are 4 types of examination risk levels. Risk is deemed negligible if the uterus is not in the primary x-ray beam and scatter radiation

Table 1
Summary of suspected in utero induced deterministic radiation effects*

Menstrual or Gestational Age	Conception Age	<50 mGy (<5 rad)	50–100 mGy (5–10 rad)	>100 mGy (>10 rad)
0–2 wk (0–14 d)	Before conception	None	None.	None.
3rd and 4th wk (15–28 d)	1st–2nd wk (1–14 d)	None	Probably none.	Possible spontaneous abortion.
5th–10th wk (29–70 d)	3rd–8th wk (15–56 d)	None	Potential effects are scientifically uncertain and probably too subtle to be clinically detectable.	Possible malformations increasing in likelihood as dose increases.
11th–17th wk (71–119 d)	9th–15th wk (57–105 d)	None	Potential effects are scientifically uncertain and probably too subtle to be clinically detectable.	Increased risk of deficits in IQ or mental retardation that increase in frequency and severity with increasing dose.
18th–27th wk (120–189 d)	16th–25th wk (106–175 d)	None	None.	IQ deficits not detectable at diagnostic doses.
>27 wk (>189 d)	>25 wk (>175 d)	None	None.	None applicable to diagnostic. medicine.

* Stochastic risks are suspected but data are not consistent [5]. For exposure to a newborn child, the lifetime risk of developing cancer is estimated on an absolute scale to be 0.4% per 10 mGy (1 rad) dose to the baby. This likely also reflects the potential risk in-utero for the second and third trimesters and part of the first trimester, but the uncertainties in this estimate are considerable.

Adapted from Zak IT, Dulai HS, Kish KK. Imaging of neurologic disorders associated with pregnancy and postpartum period. Radiographics 2007;27:95; and Kittner SJ, Stern BJ, Feeser BR, et al. Pregnancy and the risk of stroke. N Engl J Med 1996;335(11):768–74; with permission.

is too low to pose any harm; for example, head computed tomography (CT). The pelvic dose of a head CT is <0.1 mSv and shielding is no longer recommended, as it tends to cause more scatter radiation. Low-risk examinations are with fetus in the x-ray beam path but dose is well below threshold to cause developmental abnormality; for example, pelvic or lumbar spine CT (<30 mSv).[27] Examinations deemed substantial risk include multiphase abdominal and pelvic CT or CT angiogram or real-time diagnostic or therapeutic studies.

Occasionally, an examination is performed when the patient is unaware of pregnancy. The risk of these examinations is invariably negligible, as most if not all are low-risk examinations. Imaging remote from the fetus can be done safely at any time, whereas fetal doses of 100 mSv are not reached even with 3 pelvic CT or 20 conventional radiographic studies.[28] Even in situations requiring direct-beam higher-dose fluoroscopy or radiation therapy, there are options to delay examinations or tailor them to minimize exposure through technical means.[29] Advances in CT technology have resulted in better dose reduction while computer-generated CT scan parameters and dose estimates are included on every CT study to provide data and feedback for radiation safety and quality assessment purposes.[30]

There is no guideline established by the Food and Drug Administration (FDA) for MRI of fetus, as most studies did not show any associated increased risk. There is some hypothesized risk in animal and in vitro studies that include teratogenic effects and other lesser issues such as acoustic noise and heating from energy deposition.[31,32] Overall, the ACR advocates use of MR if there is need and direct benefit to the mother and fetus.

For contrast usage, iodinated contrast was shown to be mutagenic in vitro, although animal studies did not show teratogenic effect.[33] It can potentially cause neonatal hypothyroidism if introduced directly into the amniotic cavity, although currently most studies use nonionic contrast that has no effect on the thyroid gland. MR contrast agents are categorized as a Class C drug by the FDA.[34–36] Intravenous gadolinium chelate was shown to be teratogenic in animal studies (with high and repeated dose), although was not observed in a small number of human studies. Gadolinium crosses the placenta and is excreted by fetal kidneys.

In the past, cessation of breastfeeding was recommended for 24 hours after administration of contrast in a lactating mother. However, studies found that less than 0.01% of CT and 0.04% of MR contrast gets into breast milk and only a tiny fraction of ingested contrast is absorbed by the infant's gastrointestinal tract. It was thus determined that the tiny risk is not sufficient to advocate cessation of breastfeeding.[33,37–39]

To summarize, deterministic effects are negligible at any gestational age for low-risk examinations. The risks and benefits of MR are the same as without pregnancy. CT contrast is safe to use, but MR contrast be used only if necessary. There is no need to stop breastfeeding, except with the use of nuclear medicine agents. Although many imaging examinations are considered safe in pregnancy, elective imaging should be delayed and informed discussion among patient, radiologist, and medical physicist is often the most optimal course.

HEMORRHAGE

Intracranial hemorrhage during pregnancy can be caused by stroke,[40] rupture of aneurysms, or arteriovenous malformations,[41] and less frequently as sequelae from trauma, preeclampsia/eclampsia, venous thrombosis, or coagulopathy. There has been no definitive study of hemorrhage risk during pregnancy, with some suggesting slightly increased risk during the third trimester and postpartum period.[7] As in the nonpregnant population, epidural/subdural hemorrhages are seen in trauma, whereas subarachnoid hemorrhages are due to aneurysm rupture. Parenchymal hemorrhage can be seen in trauma, bleeding from vascular lesions, and hypertensive etiologies.

For acute hemorrhage, CT is the modality of choice, with low radiation risk, availability, and very short imaging time. Nonionic contrast can be administered for evaluation of vascular lesions or tumors. MR is more sensitive in detecting nonacute bleeds, acute infarcts, and small lesions or vascular abnormalities. The appearance of hemorrhage on MR is determined by the oxidized state of hemoglobin iron within or outside the erythrocyte. Signal on T1 and T2 MRIs are explained by relaxation (proximity of water protons and availability of unpaired electrons of iron) and susceptibility of hemoglobin within hematoma, respectively. Acute hemorrhage (deoxyhemoglobin) is isodense or hypodense to brain on T1, dark on T2, whereas subacute blood (methemoglobin) is bright on T1 and either bright or dark on T2 depending on being intracellular or extracellular (**Fig. 1**).

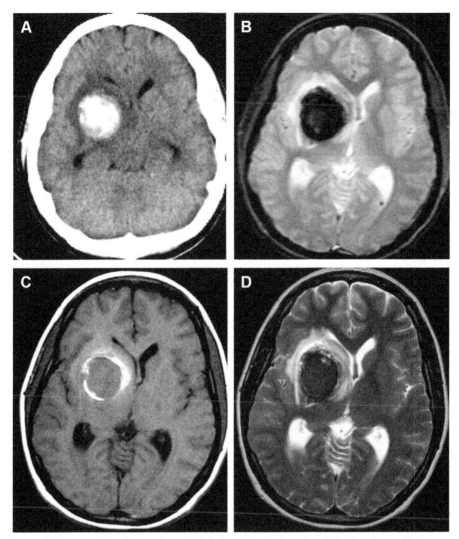

Fig. 1. A 32-year-old at 31 weeks with left hemiplegia showing right basal ganglia hemorrhage on CT (*A*), susceptibility on susceptibility-weighted imaging (SWI) (*B*), central T1 iso and T2 low signal with rim of high T1 and high T2 signal representing deoxy (*C*) and methemoglobin (*D*), respectively.

PREECLAMPSIA/ECLAMPSIA

Preeclampsia and eclampsia tend to occur during late pregnancy, extending into 6 to 8 weeks postpartum.[42] Preeclampsia is defined as new onset of hypertension and proteinuria, whereas eclampsia is preeclampsia with seizure/coma. Preeclampsia/ eclampsia is a major cause of fetal and maternal morbidity and mortality (10%–15% maternal death) with an incidence of 2% to 10%. Risk factors include age (>40), high body mass index (BMI), family history, cardiac disease, twins or multiple birth gestations, prior preeclampsia, and preexisting medical conditions, such as hypertension, insulin-dependent diabetes, or autoimmune renal disease.[43] A meta-analysis showed history of preeclampsia and presence of anti-phospholipid antibodies are the most important risk factors, whereas BMI of greater than 35, maternal age older than 40, and systemic blood pressure >130 double the risk. The use of intravenous magnesium sulfate and improved prenatal care have been credited with the decline in eclampsia for the past 20 years.[44–46] Cause of preeclampsia/eclampsia is unknown, but is thought that immune-driven superficial placenta implantation and decreased angiogenic growth factor result in utero-placental ischemia. This leads to increased placental debris in the maternal circulation eliciting inflammatory response targeting maternal endothelium. Data also suggest a 10-fold increased risk in patients with eclampsia of developing venous thrombosis and other complications, such as hemorrhage, cardiomyopathy, and amniotic fluid embolism.[47] A reported 10% of patients with preeclampsia will develop HELLP syndrome (hemolytic anemia, elevated liver enzymes, and low platelet count).[48]

Patients with preeclampsia present with headache, confusion, right upper quadrant pain, and visual disturbances, whereas those with eclampsia have seizures. They can also present with severe headache, cortical blindness, and seizure, identical to the symptoms seen in PRES/RPLS (posterior reversible encephalopathy syndrome/reversible posterior leukoencephalopathy syndrome). The etiology of PRES remains unknown, although it is thought to involve circulating substances that increase vascular permeability and disrupt cerebral autoregulation leading to vasospasm or hemorrhage.[49]

On imaging, preeclampsia/eclampsia may appear normal, although typically demonstrates symmetric subcortical white matter vasogenic edema at the parietal-occipital junction (**Fig. 2**). Despite "posterior" and "reversible" being in the names of PRES and RPLS, the imaging findings can involve anterior circulation, deep gray matter, and brainstem, and can be irreversible.

STROKE

Pregnancy and peripartum period are hypercoagulable states, due to altered hemodynamics and clotting factors, such as proteins S, C, fibrinogen, and factors VII, VIII, and X.[50] A Canadian study of strokes associated with pregnancy demonstrated an

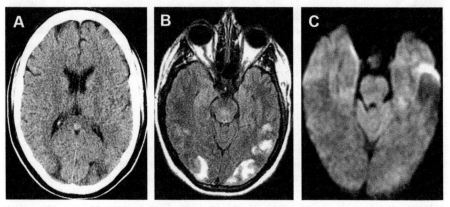

Fig. 2. A 36-year-old at 32 weeks with hypertensive episode and seizure. Bilateral symmetric low attenuation on CT (*A*) and increased signal FLAIR MR (*B*) at the parietal-occipital junction subcortical white matter without associated DWI abnormality (*C*) consistent with PRES/eclampsia.

incidence of 26 strokes per 100,000 pregnancies.[40] Most patients present in the third trimester/postpartum period with 60% due to arterial occlusions, and 40% from venous thrombosis. This elevated risk time frame may reflect labor-associated arterial dissections and large physiologic fluid shifts during delivery. Other etiologies of stroke include preeclampsia/eclampsia, postpartum cerebral angiopathy, and cardiac emboli related to various heart diseases.

Cerebral venous thrombosis also has increased incidence in the peripartum period, with greatest risk during first 2 weeks postpartum.[51] Clinical presentation varies from headache, focal neurologic deficit, altered mental status, and coma. Imaging shows high density within thrombosed sinus on noncontrast CT with "empty delta sign" filling defect within the postcontrast sinus. MR shows high signal within venous sinus on T1 sequence and blooming on gradient/susceptibility-weighted images with filling defect on postcontrast images. Venous infarcts show decreased diffusivity and/or hemorrhage often peripheral in location (**Fig. 3**).

POSTPARTUM ANGIOPATHY

Postpartum angiopathy (PPA) is a rare, reversible vasoconstriction syndrome that occurs postpartum and presents with "thunderclap" headache, focal neurologic deficits, and seizures. It is also known as Call-Fleming syndrome, although this term is more

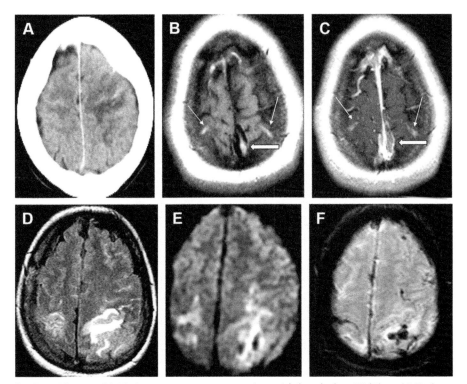

Fig. 3. A 20-year-old 10 days postpartum presenting with headache. CT (*A*) and MR shows hemorrhagic (SWI (*F*)) left greater than right venous infarcts (FLAIR (*D*), DWI (*F*)) due to cortical veins (*small arrows* [*B*, *C*]) and superior sinus thrombosis (*large arrow* [*B*, *C*]) showing short T1 signal on noncontrast (*B*) and filling defect on postcontrast images (*C*).

general and includes angiopathy occurring secondary to drugs and outside the peripartum period. Imaging features are like those of PRES. On CT angiography, MR angiography (MRA), and conventional angiogram, PPA tends to involve large and medium-sized vessels (in contrast to PRES, which usually involves more medium and small vessels) with multifocal segmental narrowing often involving anterior circulation. This vascular stenosis resolves over time and is rarely associated with infarct or hemorrhage (**Fig. 4**).[52]

NEOPLASMS

The altered hormonal balance during pregnancy can cause increase in size of preexisting CNS tumors, such as meningiomas, pituitary adenomas, schwannomas, and metastatic carcinomas. MR is superior to CT in differentiating intra-axial and extra-axial lesions, although CT can add value, as MR contrast is less indicated during pregnancy (**Figs. 5** and **6**).

In addition, there are pregnancy-specific malignancies ranging from benign to invasive molar pregnancy to choriocarcinoma. As choriocarcinoma is a highly vascular tumor, brain metastases are often hemorrhagic.[53,54]

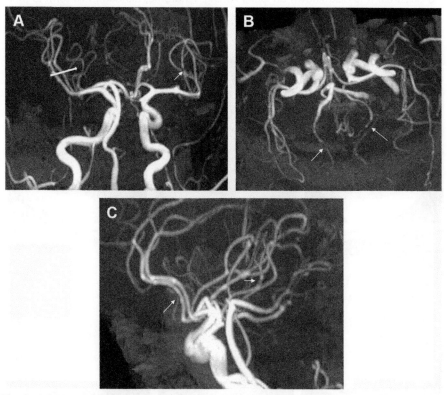

Fig. 4. A 30-year-old presenting on postpartum day 5 with severe headache. MRA of circle of Willis shows multiple focal segments of irregularity, including anterior cerebral artery (*long arrow* [*C*]), left middle cerebral artery (MCA) (*short arrow* [*B, C*]), right MCA (*long arrow* [*A*]), and bilateral posterior cerebral artery (*B*) branches suggestive of reversible cerebral vasoconstriction syndrome.

PITUITARY

The pituitary also undergoes physiologic changes during pregnancy. Rising levels of estrogen stimulate production of prolactin resulting in normal hypertrophy of adenohypophysis.[55] It reaches peak size during the first few days after delivery when it is vulnerable to infarction/hemorrhage, leading to apoplexy. This may occur within a pre-existing adenoma or hypertrophied gland itself. The patient typically has severe headache and visual disturbances.[56] On imaging, hemorrhage and decreased diffusivity may be identified within the enlarged gland (**Fig. 7**).

Pituitary apoplexy can result in Sheehan syndrome, a clinical diagnosis related to pan-hypopituitarism secondary to an episode of hypotension during delivery or the postpartum period resulting in infarction.[57] The pituitary gland is diminished in size on imaging with partial or complete empty sella.

Lymphocytic hypophysitis is a rare autoimmune process resulting in destruction of pituitary gland and endocrine deficiencies. It is estimated that approximately 50% of cases occur during late pregnancy or the early postpartum period.[58,59] In acute phase, the pituitary gland is enlarged and homogeneously enhancing with thickening of infundibulum.

WERNICKE ENCEPHALOPATHY

Wernicke encephalopathy is caused by thiamine deficiency and is most commonly associated with chronic alcoholism and malnutrition. It can be seen in pregnant patients due to excessive vomiting in the setting of hyperemesis gravidarum against a background of increased fetal thiamine demand. MR is the modality of choice demonstrating increased T2/fluid-attenuated inversion recovery (FLAIR) signal typically in mammillary bodies, thalami, periaqueductal gray, tectum, and floor of fourth ventricle. There have been reports of atypical involvement of cranial nerve nuclei and cortex in pregnant versus alcoholic patients, although remains controversial[60] (**Fig. 8**).

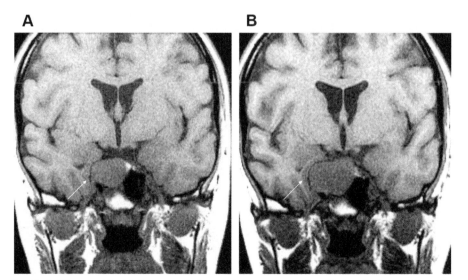

Fig. 5. A 35-year-old with known pituitary adenoma presents with headache at 34 weeks. Pre-pregnant (*A*) and pregnant (*B*) coronal T1 images show increase in size of pituitary adenoma (*arrows*).

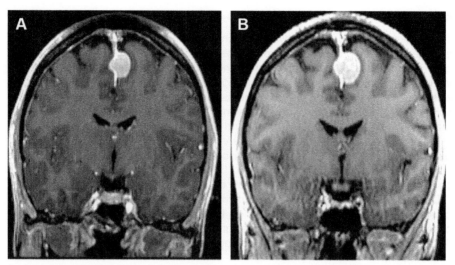

Fig. 6. A 44-year-old pre (*A*) and postpartum (*B*) coronal contrast T1 MR images show interval growth of parafalcine meningioma after more than 6 years of stability on imaging.

MULTIPLE SCLEROSIS

Multiple sclerosis is more common in women (2:1 ratio) and often occurs during reproductive age. Hormonal and immunologic effects during pregnancy are thought to result in decrease in the relapse rate, especially during the third trimester. Symptoms return to baseline or even increase up to 3 months postpartum.[9,10,61] MR again is superior to CT in detecting demyelinating lesions, typically demonstrating focal increased T2/FLAIR signal in the middle cerebellar peduncle, corpus callosum, subcortical white matter, and optic nerves. Associated enhancement indicates acute demyelination, although with advanced imaging techniques of volumetric MR and

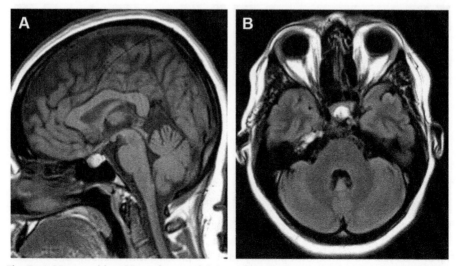

Fig. 7. A 35-year-old at 37 weeks complaining of headache. Sagittal T1 (*A*) and axial FLAIR (*B*) show increased signal within the pituitary consistent with hemorrhage and apoplexy.

diffusion-weighted imaging (DWI), contrast may not be necessary to detect most acute demyelinating lesions (**Fig. 9**).

BACK PAIN

Back pain during pregnancy can be due to increased spinal lordosis, hormonally induced ligament laxity, or pressure on lumbosacral plexus from an enlarged uterus.

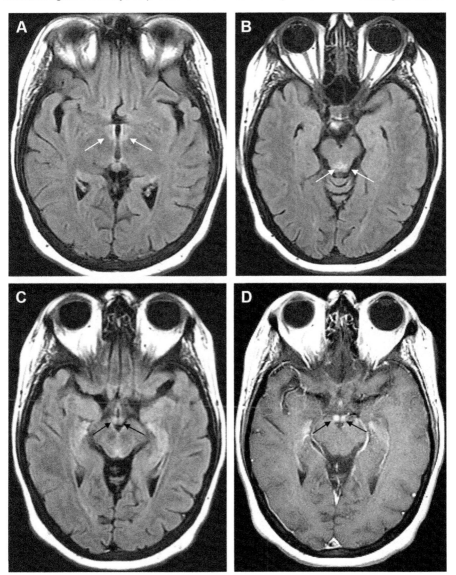

Fig. 8. A 31-year-old with history of gastric bypass with 1 month history of nausea and vomiting presenting with gait disturbance and diplopia. Figure 8 *A* and *B* both show a pair of *white arrows* pointing to abnormality and *C* and *D* shows each a pair of *black arrows*. FLAIR MR shows signal abnormality involving bilateral anterior third ventricle walls (*A*), periaqueductal gray (*B*), and mammillary bodies (*C*), the latter with associated enhancement (*D*), all consistent with Wernicke.

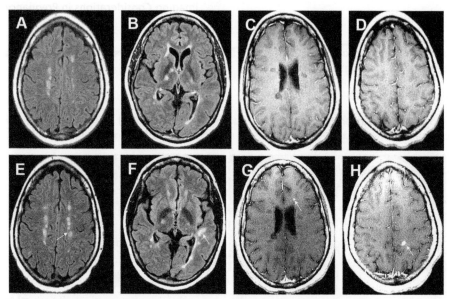

Fig. 9. A 35-year-old patient with MS showing multiple new demyelinating left periventricular and temporal white matter lesions (*arrow* [*E, F*] compared with before [*A, B*]) during first pregnancy at 22 weeks and multiple enhancing left frontal (*arrow* [*G, H*] compared with before [*C, D*]) lesions 2 weeks postpartum after second pregnancy.

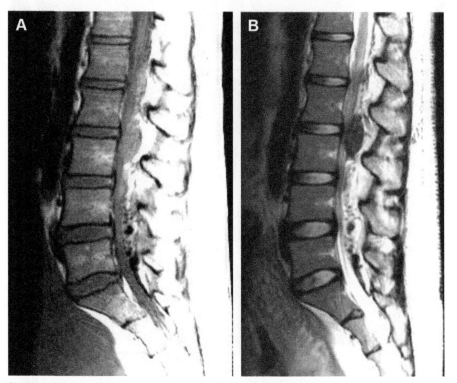

Fig. 10. A 30-year-old who had epidural catheter placed for labor presents with back pain and right lower extremity weakness 2 days postpartum. Sagittal MR T1 (*A*) and T2 (*B*) images of the lumbar spine show a heterogenous collection of hemorrhage at different stages at the posterior epidural space causing canal stenosis from L1-2 to L5 worst at L2-3 level.

MR is the modality of choice for evaluation of disc disease and epidural or paraspinal processes, such as infection, hematoma, or preexisting spinal tumors. Cauda equina syndrome secondary to disc extrusion has been reported in 1 of 10,000 births.[62] Epidural hematoma can result spontaneously from increased intra-abdominal pressure during delivery or rarely as a complication from epidural anesthesia[63] **(Fig. 10)**. As with intracranial tumors, hormonal effects can have a trophic effect on spine tumors, which may become symptomatic during pregnancy.[64] T1, T2, and if needed postcontrast MR images are helpful in delineating and differentiating epidural, subdural, and intramedullary processes.

SUMMARY

There are many situations during pregnancy in which imaging is necessary for diagnosis and treatment. Although most diagnostic imaging is low risk to the mother and fetus, one should always weigh the risks and benefits on a case-by-case basis. Knowledge and understanding of imaging findings and appropriate selection of the optimal modality facilitates prompt diagnosis and treatment while minimizing potential harm to mother and fetus.

REFERENCES

1. Royek AB, Parisi VM. Maternal biological adaptations to pregnancy. In: Hobbins JC, Reece EA, editors. Medicine of the fetus and mother. Philadelphia: Lippincott-Raven; 1999. p. 903–20.
2. Oatridge A, Holdcroft A, Saeed N, et al. Change in brain size during and after pregnancy: study in healthy women and women with preeclampsia. AJNR Am J Neuroradiol 2002;23:19–26.
3. Zak IT, Dulai HS, Kish KK. Imaging of neurologic disorders associated with pregnancy and postpartum period. Radiographics 2007;27:95.
4. Kittner SJ, Stern BJ, Feeser BR, et al. Pregnancy and the risk of stroke. N Engl J Med 1996;335(11):768–74.
5. Wilterdink JL, Feldmann E. Intracranial hemorrhage. Adv Neurol 2002;90:63–74.
6. Stoodley MA, Macdonald RL, Weir BK. Pregnancy and intracranial aneurysms. Neurosurg Clin N Am 1998;9:549.
7. Bateman BT, Schumacher HC, Bushnell CD, et al. Intracerebral hemorrhage in pregnancy: frequency, risk factors, and outcome. Neurology 2006;67(3):424–9.
8. Leber A, teles A, zenclussen AC. Regulatory T cells and their role in pregnancy. Am J Reprod Immunol 2010;63:445–59.
9. Confavreux C, Hutchinson M, Hours MM, et al. Rate of pregnancy related relapse in multiple sclerosis. N Engl J Med 1998;339:285–91.
10. Vukusic S, Hutchinson M, Hours M, et al. For the pregnancy in multiple sclerosis group: pregnancy and multiple sclerosis (the PRIMS study): clinical predictors of postpartum relapse. Brain 2004;127:1353–60.
11. International Commission on Radiological Protection publication 84: paragraph 12.
12. Background rad United Nations Scientific Committee on the Effects of Atomic Radiation. Sources and effects of ionizing radiation. New York: United Nations (published 2010); 2008. p. 4.
13. Occupation exposure "The 2007 recommendations of the International Commission on Radiological Protection. ICRP publication 103". Ann ICRP 2007;37(2–4): 1–332.
14. Aviation National Council on Radiation Protection and measurements report 160. Available at: https://ncrponline.org/publications/reports/ncrp-report-160.

15. Acute radiation syndrome: a fact sheet for physicians. Centers for Disease Control and Prevention; 2005. Available at: https://emergency.cdc.gov/radiation/pdf/prenatal.pdf.
16. Russell LB, Russell WL. An analysis of the changing radiation response of the developing mouse embryo. J Cell Physiol Suppl 1954;43(Suppl. 1):103–49.
17. Yamazaki JN, Schull WJ. Perinatal loss and neurological abnormalities among children of the atomic bomb. Nagasaki and Hiroshima revisited, 1949 to 1989. JAMA 1990;264(5):605–9.
18. Dekaban AS. Abnormalities in children exposed to x-radiation during various stages of gestation: tentative timetable of radiation injury to the human fetus. I. J Nucl Med 1968;9(9):471–7.
19. Stewart A, Kneale GW. Radiation dose effects in relation to obstetric x-rays and childhood cancers. Lancet 1970;1(7658):1185–8.
20. American College of Radiology (ACR). ACR guidelines and technical standards. Practice guideline for imaging pregnant or potentially pregnant adolescents and women with ionizing radiation. 1st edition. Reston (VA): American College of Radiology; 2008. p. 1–15.
21. Hall EJ, Giaccia AJ. Radiobiology for the radiologist. Philadelphia: Lippincott, Williams, and Wilkins; 2006 j34.
22. Osei EK, Faulkner K. Fetal doses from radiological examinations. Br J Radiol 1999;72(860):773–80.
23. International Commission on Radiological Protection publication 84: paragraph 22.
24. Wakeford R, Little MP. Risk coefficients for childhood cancer after intrauterine irradiation. Int J Radiat Biol 2003;79:293–309.
25. International Commission on Radiological Protection publication 84: paragraph 22-40.
26. International Commission on Radiological Protection publication 84: paragraph 73.
27. Huda W, Randazzo W, Tipnis S, et al. Embryo dose estimates in body CT. AJR Am J Roentgenol 2010;194:874–80.
28. International Commission on Radiological Protection publication 84: paragraph 25.
29. International Commission on Radiological Protection publication 84: paragraph 58, 64.
30. Kaza RK, Platt JF, Al-Hawary MM, et al. CT enterography at 80 kVp with adaptive statistical iterative reconstruction versus at 120 kVp with standard reconstruction: image quality, diagnostic adequacy and dose reduction. AJR Am J Roentgenol 2012;198:1084–92.
31. Yip YP, Capriotti C, Talagala SL, et al. Effects of MR exposure at 1.5 T on early embryonic development of the chick. J Magn Reson Imaging 1994;4(5):742–8.
32. Kanal E, Shellock FG, Talagala L. Safety considerations in MR imaging. Radiology 1990;176(3):593–606.
33. Webb JA, Thomsen HS, Morcos SK. Members of Contrast Media Safety Committee of European Society of Urogenital Radiology (ESUR). The use of iodinated and gadolinium contrast media during pregnancy and lactation. Eur Radiol 2005;15(6):1234–40.
34. Rodesch F, Camus M, Ermans AM, et al. Adverse effect of amniofetography on fetal thyroid function. Am J Obstet Gynecol 1976;126(6):723–6.
35. Bona G, Zaffaroni M, Defilippi C, et al. Effects of iopamidol on neonatal thyroid function. Eur J Radiol 1992;14(1):22–5.

36. Gruters A, Krude H. Detection and treatment of congenital hypothyroidism. Nat Rev Endocrinol 2011;8:104–13.
37. American College of Radiology. ACR practice guideline for the use of intravascular contrast media. Reston (VA): American College of Radiology; 2007. p. 1–6.
38. Kanal E, Barkovich AJ, Bell C. ACR blue ribbon panel on MR safety et al. ACR guidance document for safe MR practices: 2007. AJR Am J Roentgenol 2007; 188(6).1447–74.
39. Nelson JA, Livingston GK, Moon RG. Mutagenic evaluation of radiographic contrast media. Invest Radiol 1982;17(2):183–5.
40. Jaigobin C, Silver FL. Stroke and pregnancy. Stroke 2000;31:2948–51.
41. Dias MS, Sekhar LN. Intracranial hemorrhage from aneurysms and arteriovenous malformations during pregnancy and the puerperium. Neurosurgery 1990;27: 855–65.
42. Duckitt K, Harrington D. Risk factors for pre-eclampsia at antenatal booking: a systematic review of controlled studies. BMJ 2005;330:565–7.
43. Liu S, Joseph KS, Liston RM, et al. Incidence, risk factors, and associated complications of eclampsia. Obstet Gynecol 2011;118(5):987–94.
44. Fong A, Chau CT, Pan D, et al. Clinical morbidities, trends, and demographics of eclampsia: a population-based study. Am J Obstet Gynecol 2013;209(3):e1–7.
45. O'Connor HD, Hehir MP, Kent EM, et al. Eclampsia: trends in incidence and outcomes over 30 years. Am J Perinatol 2013;30:661–4.
46. Altman D, Carroli G, Duley L, et al. Do women with pre-eclampsia, and their babies, benefit from magnesium sulphate? The Magpie trial: a randomized placebo-controlled trial. Lancet 2002;359:1877–90.
47. Bates SM, Greer IA, Middeldorp S, et al. VTE, thrombophilia, antithrombotic therapy, and pregnancy: antithrombotic therapy and prevention of thrombosis, 9th ed: American College of Chest Physicians evidence-based clinical practice guidelines. Chest 2012;141:e691S–736S.
48. Takahashi K, Ohkuchi A, Kobayashi M, et al. Recurrence risk of hypertensive disease in pregnancy. Med J Obstet Gynecol 2014;2(2):1023, p1-6.
49. Bartynski WS. Posterior reversible encephalopathy syndrome, part 2: controversies surrounding pathophysiology of vasogenic edema. AJNR Am J Neuroradiol 2008;29(6):1043–9.
50. Comeglio P, Fedi S, Liotta AA, et al. Blood clotting activation during normal pregnancy. Thromb Res 1996;84(3):199–202.
51. Mas JL, Lamy C. Stroke in pregnancy and the puerperium. J Neurol 1998; 245(6–7):305–13.
52. Ducros A. Reversible cerebral vasoconstriction syndrome. Handb Clin Neurol 2014;121:1725–41.
53. Altieri A, Franceschi S, Ferlay J, et al. Epidemiology and aetiology of gestational trophoblastic diseases. Lancet Oncol 2003;4:670–8.
54. Huang CY, Chen CA, Hsieh CY, et al. Intracerebral hemorrhage as initial presentation of gestational choriocarcinoma: a case report and literature review. Int J Gynecol Cancer 2007;17:1166–71.
55. Foyouzi N, Frisbaek Y, Norwitz ER. Pituitary gland and pregnancy. Obstet Gynecol Clin North Am 2004;31(4):873–92, xi.
56. Shimon I. Clinical features of pituitary apoplexy. In: Turgut M, Mahapatra AK, Powell M, et al, editors. Pituitary apoplexy. Berlin: Springer-Verlag; 2014. p. 49–54.
57. Keleştimur F. Sheehan's syndrome. Pituitary 2003;6(4):181–8.

58. Ahmadi J, Meyers GS, Segall HD, et al. Lymphocytic adenohypophysitis: contrast-enhanced MR imaging in five cases. Radiology 1995;195(1):30–4.
59. Kanekar S, Bennett S. Imaging of neurologic conditions in pregnant patients. Radiographics 2016;36(7):2102–22.
60. Manzo G, De Gennaro A, Cozzolino A, et al. MR imaging findings in alcoholic and nonalcoholic acute Wernicke's encephalopathy: a review. Biomed Res Int 2014; 2014:503576.
61. Soldan SS, Alvarez Retuerto AI, Sicotte NL, et al. Immune modulation in multiple sclerosis patients treated with the pregnancy hormone estriol. J Immunol 2003; 171(11):6267–74.
62. LaBan MM, Perrin JC, Latimer FR. Pregnancy and herniated lumbar disc. Arch Phys Med Rehabil 1983;64:319–21.
63. Yonekawa Y, Mehdorn HM, Nishikawa M. Spontaneous spinal epidural hematoma during pregnancy. Surg Neurol 1975;3(6):327–8.
64. Kiroglu Y, Benel B, Yagci B, et al. Spinal cord compression caused by vertebral hemangioma being symptomatic during pregnancy. Surg Neurol 2009;71: 487–92.

Management of Demyelinating Disorders in Pregnancy

Tamara B. Kaplan, MD

KEYWORDS

- Multiple sclerosis • Neuromyelitis optica • Demyelinating disease • Relapse
- Disease-modifying therapy • Pregnancy • Lactation

KEY POINTS

- Multiple sclerosis (MS) is a female-predominate disease that often first presents during a women's childbearing years.
- Women with MS should be counseled early and often on reproduction, pregnancy planning, and length of time needed off disease-modifying medications before attempting conception.
- Pregnancy appears to be protective against MS disease activity, particularly during the second and third trimesters, with an increased risk of relapse in the first 3 months postpartum.
- Women with MS who want to have children should be supported and encouraged to do so.
- Women with neuromyelitis optica spectrum disorder are vulnerable to both postpartum relapses and relapses during pregnancy. In addition, they are at higher risk for other pregnancy complications, such as miscarriage and preeclampsia.

INTRODUCTION

Multiple sclerosis (MS) is a chronic demyelinating disease of the central nervous system (CNS). MS affects twofold to threefold more women than men, and the disease often first presents during peak childbearing years.[1] Historically, women with MS were advised against pregnancy,[2] but more recently, it appears that pregnancy is a benign event in the course of MS. Within the past 2 decades, consistent attempts have been made to study this issue via retrospective and prospective analyses.[3,4] Additionally, new data on safety and efficacy of immunomodulating MS treatments for pregnant and lactating women are continually emerging.

Department of Neurology, Partners Multiple Sclerosis Center, Brigham and Women's Hospital, Harvard Medical School, 60 Fenwood Road, 4th Floor, Boston, MA 02115, USA
E-mail address: tbkaplan@bwh.harvard.edu

Neurol Clin 37 (2019) 17–30
https://doi.org/10.1016/j.ncl.2018.09.007
0733-8619/19/© 2018 Elsevier Inc. All rights reserved.

Neuromyelitis optica spectrum disorder (NMOSD) is also a female-predominant disease[5,6] that often affects women during their childbearing years,[7] but the course of disease during pregnancy differs from MS.

EFFECTS OF PREGNANCY ON MULTIPLE SCLEROSIS DISEASE COURSE
Antepartum and Postpartum Effects

There was a major shift in thinking regarding pregnancy in MS with the landmark 1998 Pregnancy in Multiple Sclerosis (PRIMS) study, which is the best large-scale prospective study published. PRIMS enrolled 254 women (246 with relapsing MS), and 269 pregnancies, and patients were followed for at least 12 months postpartum. Compared with prepregnancy, annualized relapse rate fell by 70% during the third trimester. However, during the first 3 months postpartum, the relapse rate increased to 70% above the prepregnancy level, and eventually returned to the prepregnancy rate after those initial 3 months. The annualized relapse rate from postpartum months 3 to 12 was not significantly different from that of the prepregnancy year.[3] In a follow-up study, clinical predictors of a likelihood of postpartum relapse in PRIMS were evaluated. Three variables correlated significantly with the occurrence of a postpartum relapse[4]: increased relapse rate in the year before pregnancy, increased relapse rate during pregnancy and higher Expanded Disability Status Scale score at the onset of pregnancy. Epidural anesthesia and breastfeeding were not predictive of a postpartum relapse or of disability progression. The findings of the PRIMS study have been replicated by numerous other studies since its initial publication.[8,9]

Long-Term Effects

The precise effects of childbearing on long-term disability progression in MS are unclear, but overall, it appears that pregnancy does not seem to worsen disease and disability. A prospective 5-year study compared rates of disability progression among childless women, women who had onset of MS after childbirth, and women who had onset before or during pregnancy. The rates of disability increased most rapidly in nulliparous women.[10] However, another retrospective population-based study of 185 women with MS found no association between disability and total number of term pregnancies, timing of pregnancy relative to disease onset, or either onset or worsening of MS in relation to a pregnancy.[11] Importantly, results of such studies may be confounded by patient choice; women with worse disability may be more likely to choose not to become pregnant. Further prospective studies are needed to clarify the long-term effects of pregnancy on MS disease course.

APPROACH TO THE PATIENT WITH MULTIPLE SCLEROSIS PLANNING PREGNANCY

Overall, fertility does not seem to be impaired in women with MS,[12] but some studies have investigated whether subtle hormonal imbalances in patients with MS may perhaps contribute to reduced fertility.[13–15] Clinicians can reassure patients that, in most studies, there does not appear to be an increase in spontaneous abortions, stillbirths, cesarean deliveries, premature births, or birth defects in mothers with MS.[16]

Vitamin D

In addition to taking prenatal vitamins and folic acid and avoiding alcohol and smoking, women with MS should be encouraged to take vitamin D. Low vitamin D levels are thought to be a risk factor for the development of MS.[17] Furthermore, low maternal vitamin D during pregnancy may potentially increase the risk of developing MS among offspring.[18] Although vitamin D is certainly important, the ideal serum levels for patients with MS who are pregnant or trying to conceive are unknown. Currently, the American College of Obstetrics and Gynecology does not recommend routine screening in all pregnant women, and notes that 1000 to 2000 IU per day of vitamin D is safe for those who are deficient.[19] Vitamin D levels should be checked in women with MS who are pregnant or trying to conceive, and they should supplement accordingly.

Assisted Reproductive Technology

Some women may choose to use assisted reproductive technology (ART) in effort to conceive. Several small, heterogeneous studies have reported an increase in relapse rate in the 3-month period following use of ART, especially if gonadotropin-releasing hormone agonists were used and if the cycle was unsuccessful.[12,20–25] However, these studies do not adequately account for the effects of disease-modifying therapy (DMT) interruption on inflammatory activity. Larger prospective studies are clearly needed to better understand this potential concern.

MANAGEMENT OF MULTIPLE SCLEROSIS DURING PREGNANCY
Treating Relapse During Pregnancy

Although relapses are less common in pregnancy, they may still occur, especially in the first 2 trimesters, and should be managed appropriately. If imaging is warranted, MRI is likely safe. There are no conclusive data to show that MRI exposure up to 3 T is associated with fetal harm, but gadolinium should be avoided in pregnancy.[26] Gadolinium can enter fetal circulation and in animal studies, high doses of gadolinium were associated with miscarriage and developmental abnormalities.[26] New lesions suggestive of a relapse can be visualized on MRI without gadolinium, if a baseline scan is available for comparison. If a relapse is severe enough to warrant therapy, methylprednisolone is the preferred steroid, as it is metabolized before crossing the placenta. For many years, it was thought that steroid use during the first trimester increased risk of cleft palate.[27–29] However, 2 recent studies, the National Birth Defect Prevention Study,[30] and a large Danish prevalence study, observed no associated risk of cleft lip/palate or other congenital malformations in offspring of more than a thousand women who used inhaled or oral corticosteroids through the first trimester.[31] In addition, intravenous immunoglobulin (IVIg) therapy is safe to use during pregnancy, has a very low rate of maternal side effects, and no known negative influence on the developing fetal immune system. Studies suggest that IVIg may help prevent MS relapses both during pregnancy and postpartum.[32]

Disease-Modifying Therapies During Pregnancy

The US Food and Drug Administration (FDA) has now approved more than 15 DMTs for the treatment of relapsing forms of MS, and 1 has been approved for primary progressive MS. Per the FDA and the National MS Society consensus statements, DMTs should not be used in patients with MS who are pregnant, trying to conceive, or breastfeeding (https://www.nationalmssociety.org/Living-Well-With-MS/Diet-Exercise-Healthy-Behaviors/Womens-Health/Pregnancy). In practice, there is wide variability of practice patterns relating to DMT discontinuation before conception.[33] Choosing when to stop a DMT before conception can be a difficult decision for many women with MS. Although there may be potential risks of conceiving while on a DMT, there also may be a risk of relapse if therapy is held too long. When the objective is complete elimination before conception, a period of 5 maximal half-lives is recommended, except for teriflunomide, which requires a specific washout protocol. Based on this principle, for DMTs with shorter half-lives (**Table 1**), such as interferon β, glatiramer acetate, and dimethyl fumarate, a short washout period is likely sufficient, but longer washout periods are required for the other oral and infusion DMTs.[34]

Finally, many pregnancies may be unintentional, and thus, it is imperative that clinicians engage in pregnancy counseling with all women of reproductive age to inform them of the potential risks of conception on various DMTs. These effects are summarized in **Table 1**.

Interferons (betaseron, rebif, avonex, extavia, plegridy)

Interferon βs (IFN-β) are the oldest class of DMTs. There is no animal evidence of teratogenicity, and the large macromolecule is unlikely to cross the placenta in any significant amount. Some reports suggest maternal IFN-β exposure is associated with lower infant birth weights and higher incidence of premature births.[35–37] However, these studies all had significant limitations,[38] and more recent studies do not confirm these findings,[34,39] including a prospective cohort study from the German Multiple Sclerosis and Pregnancy Registry, which involved 251 pregnancies in mothers treated with IFN-β1a.[38] In addition, postmarketing cohort studies have shown that the risk of spontaneous abortion on IFN-β1a is not significantly different from the general population.[40] If conception occurs during use of IFN-β, there is no data-driven reason to support pregnancy termination.[41]

Table 1
Summary of effects of disease-modifying therapies on multiple sclerosis

Immunomodulating Agents	Drug Half-Life	Fetal and Maternal Risks
Interferon β-1-b and β-1-a	10 h	Spontaneous abortions in animals; not seen in humans
Glatiramer acetate	6.76 h	None reported
Intravenous immunoglobulin	25–32 d	Probably safe in pregnancy
Fingolimod	6–9 d	Teratogenicity seen in animals and humans; no specific pattern observed
Dimethyl fumarate	1 h	Increased spontaneous abortion in animals; not reported in humans
Teriflunomide	18–19 d	Teratogenicity seen in animals; precursor leflunomide is a known human teratogen; no malformations in humans observed thus far
Natalizumab	7–15 d	Reduce neonatal survival at supratherapeutic doses in primates; transient hematologic abnormalities in late pregnancy exposure in humans
Alemtuzumab	12 d	Increased rates of fetal loss, decreased B and T lymphocytes in offspring in animals; no human malformations seen, but thyroid monitoring necessary for mother throughout pregnancy; no evidence for spontaneous abortion or birth defects
Rituximab/ Ocrelizumab	22 days/26 d	No human malformations seen; transient B-cell depletion in human neonates and animals following pregnancy exposure

Glatiramer Acetate (Copaxone)

Glatiramer acetate (GA) is the only DMT with a former FDA "category B," and overall, no major concerns have been raised with GA use during pregnancy. Thus far, in more than 500 human pregnancies, GA use has shown no association with low birth weight, congenital anomaly, preterm birth, or spontaneous abortion.[40,42–44] GA is not believed to cross the placenta nor does it have measurable blood levels in the mother.[42] Currently, some neurologists treat women with GA during pregnancy.

Dimethyl Fumarate (Tecfidera)

Despite a few concerning animal studies, no significant adverse effects have been detected with human pregnancies. Animal studies showed that dimethyl fumarate (DMF), at doses 2 times higher than the approved human dose, was associated with embryo lethality in rats.[34] Additionally, when given at a dose equivalent to 16 times the normal human therapeutic dose, there was an increased spontaneous abortion rate in rabbits.[45] However, in humans, in a case series of 45 women exposed to DMT in early pregnancy, no significant adverse effects were noted. Overall, postmarketing studies of human pregnancy exposures to date have not detected any signal of elevated fetal abnormalities after first trimester exposure.[46] DMF has a very short half-life (less than 60 minutes), and therefore a short washout or no washout is currently recommended.

Fingolimod (Gilenya)

Fingolimod does cross the placenta, and in animal studies, there is evidence for both teratogenicity and embryolethality (including ventricular septal defect, persistent truncus arteriosus, Tetralogy of Fallot, acrania, malformation of the tibia, and fetal death). In a limited number of human pregnancies, there seems to be a slightly higher rate of both spontaneous abortions and malformations.[47] In 66 human exposure cases, there was a reported 7.6% rate of fetal abnormalities at birth.[48] In the fingolimod clinical trial program, among 34 pregnancies, there were 13 healthy infants, 1 with a tibia malformation (thought to be unrelated to treatment), 5 spontaneous abortions, 9 elective abortions, and 6 ongoing pregnancies at the time of publication.[49] Currently, it is recommended that fingolimod be discontinued at least 2 months before conceiving (half-life is approximately 9 days).[50] After fingolimod discontinuation, there is also concern for potential rebound disease activity,[51] and often bridging therapies are considered.

Teriflunomide (Aubagio)

Teriflunomide must be discontinued and eliminated from the body before conception.[52] Teriflunomide is the active metabolite of leflunomide, which has long been used to treat rheumatoid arthritis. Even at lower than human therapeutic doses, leflunomide has shown teratogenic and embryo lethal effects in multiple animal species.[53] Leflunomide has caused fetal abnormalities, including craniofacial, axial, and appendicular skeletal malformations in pregnant rats and rabbits. Despite these findings, of the recorded human pregnancies with exposure to teriflunomide, the rate of spontaneous abortion was not different from the general population, and no serious malformations were reported.[54]

Importantly, teriflunomide may persist in the body for as long as 24 months, even though the mean half-life is 16 to 18 days. Conception should occur only once teriflunomide levels are lower than 0.02 µg/mL. If an unplanned pregnancy occurs, or if the patient desires pregnancy within 1 year of treatment, a rapid elimination protocol with oral cholestyramine or activated charcoal over several days is used to lower teriflunomide levels to less than 0.02 µg/mL.[48] In addition to its ability to cross the placenta, teriflunomide is also present in the semen of men taking the drug.[55]

Natalizumab (Tysabri)

Natalizumab is a humanized monoclonal antibody against the cell adhesion molecule α4-integrin. Natalizumab likely does not cross into fetal circulation until the placenta is established (approximately 13–14 weeks' gestation). In animal studies, suprathera-peutic doses of natalizumab have been shown to decrease fertility and reduce neonatal survival. This medication has also been shown to cause transient hematolog-ic abnormalities in primates following maternal exposure. In humans, according to the Tysabri Pregnancy Exposure Registry, which reported 375 human pregnancies, resulting in 314 live births, the rates of miscarriage and malformation were similar to the general population. However, mild to moderate hematologic alterations, such as thrombocytopenia and anemia, have been reported in 75% of newborns who were exposed to natalizumab after the 30th gestational week.[56] Natalizumab also was detected in the cord blood of 5 of 5 newborns tested.[56]

Rebound disease activity after natalizumab withdrawal is well described, and there has been concern this may occur during pregnancy. A recent prospective case series of 40 women receiving natalizumab during pregnancy observed that newborns had fewer hematologic abnormalities when exposed to natalizumab for both less than 24 and 30 weeks' gestation, but there were significantly more relapses in the women who discontinued therapy before 24 weeks' gestation.[56,57] Based on these findings, in women with highly active disease, it may be reasonable to withdraw natalizumab at approximately 30 weeks' gestation, in the interest of both maternal and child health, as long as the newborn is evaluated for hematologic abnormalities or other complica-tions shortly after birth.[56]

Rituximab (Rituxan)/Ocrelizumab (Ocrevus)

Over the past few years, rituximab, a chimeric anti-CD20 monoclonal antibody, has been used as off-label treatment for MS.[58] Ocrelizumab, a humanized anti-CD20 anti-body, was approved by the FDA in March 2017 for treatment of both relapsing and pri-mary progressive forms of MS. Given its recent entry into the market, most of what we know about anti-CD20 therapy comes from experience with rituximab.

Rituximab is thought to cross the placenta in both animals and humans[59]; however, these studies showed no evidence of increased risk of miscarriage or teratogenicity. Transient newborn B-cell depletion has been seen in exposed animal and human pregnancies.[60] The risk of B-cell depletion in the newborn appears to be higher when the mother is exposed to the drug during the second or third trimester. Accord-ing to the current Ocrelizumab Product Information, the current recommendation is for women to use contraception while on treatment and to wait for 6 months after the last infusion before conceiving.[61]

Alemtuzumab (Lemtrada)

Alemtuzumab is an anti-CD52 humanized monoclonal antibody that is administered annually, and is typically used in patients with aggressive or refractory MS. In animal studies, early maternal administration of alemtuzumab resulted in increased rates of fetal loss as well as decreased B and T lymphocytes in offspring at birth.[34] In humans, as of 2015, 167 pregnancy outcomes were documented from the clinical development program, including 16 ongoing pregnancies and 10 women lost to follow-up. The completed pregnancies reflect the expected range of pregnancy outcomes in the gen-eral population: 110 live births with healthy neonates, 37 (22.2%) spontaneous abor-tions, 19 elective terminations, and one stillbirth.[62] Currently, women are advised to avoid conception for at least 4 months after their last infusion, even though plasma concentrations of the drug approach zero, 30 days after the last infusion.[34,63] One reason for this is the concern for possible secondary autoimmune thyroid disease in the patient and the potential effects on the unborn fetus. Maternal thyroid-stimulating hormone receptor antibodies can pass the placenta and cause transient neonatal Graves disease.[62] Pregnant women and those considering pregnancy with alemtuzumab exposure should have their thyroid function tested and monitored, as such abnormalities are a known complication of alemtuzumab therapy.[62]

Breastfeeding

Several studies suggest that breastfeeding may influence postpartum relapse rate, but the true effect continues to be debated. Some studies have reported an association between breastfeeding and decreased relapses.[64,65] However, other studies,[66] including the PRIMS cohort,[3] showed no association between breastfeeding and postpartum relapse rate or disability. Some of these differences may be due to the broad variability in breastfeeding practices in intensity, frequency, duration, and degree of supplementation. A meta-analysis reported that overall, women with MS who breastfeed were almost half as likely to experience a postpartum relapse compared with women who did not. However, the pooled analysis is limited by the confounding factor, maternal choice; women who chose to breastfeed were less likely to be using a DMT before pregnancy, likely had more benign disease activity during pregnancy, and overall and had less severe forms of MS.[67] It is likely that although women who breastfeed appear to do better, they may be preselected as having milder disease. Further research is needed to assess to true effect of postpartum disease and MRI activity.

Although there are still many questions, the available evidence suggests that breastfeeding is safe and possibly beneficial for patients with MS. Breastfeeding mothers are generally advised not to start DMT until breastfeeding is discontinued, as there are incomplete data available on the potential effects on newborns. However, we do have some information about the transfer of various DMTs into milk from animal studies and small case series.

Disease-modifying therapies and breastfeeding	
Interferons	• Not generally excreted in breast milk due to large protein size and remains in bound state with low plasma levels in the mother. • Small study reported breast milk contained only 0.006% of maternal dose of IFNβ-1a.[68] • IFNβ not orally bioavailable. • Study of 6 nursing mothers using IFN-β1a showed no side effects in infants.[69] • Levels in breastmilk are minuscule; many neurologists feel it is safe with breastfeeding.
Glatiramer acetate	• No adverse events reported in 9 mothers who breastfed their infants for mean of 3.6 months while taking GA.[42] • GA is unlikely transmitted in breast milk, but there are no definitive studies. • Even if some drug crosses into breast milk, given large molecular weight, it is likely degraded in infant's gastrointestinal tract with oral ingestion. • GA may be considered safe with breastfeeding.[70]
Dimethyl fumarate	• Active drug component in DMF, monomethyl fumarate, has low molecular weight. (129 Da) and low protein binding (27%–45%); consequently, a significant amount is thought to enter milk.[71] • At this time, lactation should be avoided when using DMF.

(continued on next page)

(continued)	
Fingolimod	• Drug is present in breast milk of rodents and is orally bioavailable.
	• No human studies, but given high volume of distribution and high protein binding,[71] levels in human milk are likely low.
	• At this time, breastfeeding should be avoided, as even small amounts transmitted in breast milk would be orally available to the infant.
Teriflunomide	• Teriflunomide has been detected in rat milk following a single dose.[50]
	• Although human data are limited, use of teriflunomide is contraindicated with breastfeeding.
Natalizumab	• Natalizumab has been detected in breast milk.
	• Although half-life is 7 to 15 days, time to reach steady state is approximately 28 weeks, so actual concentration in breast milk at steady state is still uncertain.[71]
	• Concentrations in milk may increase over time with subsequent infusions.[72]
	• Even if some drug is transmitted in breast milk, it is unclear how much would be absorbed through infant's gastrointestinal mucosa.
	• Further research is needed to evaluate any potential risk to the infant.
	• Natalizumab should not be used in lactating women at this time.
Rituximab/ Ocrelizumab	• Low levels of rituximab detected in breast milk of primates.[73]
	• Excretion of maternal immunoglobulin G antibodies into human breast milk is limited; comprise only approximately 2% of total immunoglobulin content,[74] and much of that is likely degraded in the infant's gastrointestinal system.[74]
	• Single case report found breast milk contained only 0.36% of the amount in mother's serum, suggesting minimal excretion into milk.[75]
	• No case reports have been published regarding ocrelizumab levels in breast milk, but it is reasonable to assume similar results.
	• Women treated with rituximab and ocrelizumab are typically advised not to breastfeed given a lack of human data, but further studies are needed.
Alemtuzumab	• Alemtuzumab is present in milk of lactating mice.[34]
	• Due to large molecular weight (150 kD), it is unlikely to enter breast milk in any significant amount.[71]
	• Given lack of human data and risk of potential side effects, caution should be used in breastfeeding mothers.

Management of Postpartum Relapses

Steroids and intravenous immunoglobulin

Both steroids and IVIg can be used to treat postpartum relapses and prevent relapses in women who choose to breastfeed. Pulses of monthly intravenous methylprednisolone (IVMP) may play a role in prevention of relapses. One study showed a decreased rate of relapses in women who received monthly IVMP compared with untreated women, but there was no difference in overall neurologic function or progression of disease between those treated and controls.[76] Use of IV steroids for relapse prevention in the postpartum period should be considered on an individual basis.

Historically women were advised to stop breastfeeding and "pump and dump" after receiving IV steroids, due to possible excretion into breast milk. In serial sampling of breast milk from a mother with MS who was receiving IV methylprednisolone, breast milk concentrations of methylprednisolone were highest 1 hour after steroid administration and then quickly tapered off.[77] Another study showed that even when the mother received large doses of steroids, the amount ingested by the infant was only between 1.1% and 1.5% of maternal dose. This is well below the accepted relative infant dose of 10% for medications excreted into breast milk and far less than any therapeutic dose of steroids for an infant.[69] However, if the mother wishes to limit infant exposure even further, she could wait 2 to 4 hours after receiving IVMP, which will significantly reduce the amount of drug in her milk.

Breastfeeding is not contraindicated during IVIg therapy. A pilot study of 104 patients reported a lower rate of postpartum relapses in patients treated with IVIg. Significant postpartum relapse rate reduction ($P<.05$) was observed in patients who received IVIg continuously throughout pregnancy and until 12 weeks postpartum.[78] Other studies have also suggested that postpartum administration of IVIg could be beneficial in preventing relapses during this period.[79]

NEUROMYELITIS OPTICA SPECTRUM DISORDERS IN PREGNANCY

Neuromyelitis optica (NMO), now termed neuromyelitis optica spectrum disorder (NMOSD), is a relapsing, inflammatory neurologic disease that primarily effects the optic nerves and spinal cord. NMOSD is female-predominant (7–9 F:1 M),[5,6] more common in nonwhite populations,[6,80] and often affects women during their childbearing years.[7] Approximately 68% to 91% of patients are seropositive for pathogenic antibodies targeting Aquaporin-4 (AQP4–immunoglobulin G [IgG]), and seropositivity appears more frequent in women.[81] The water channel, AQP4, is most greatly expressed on the foot processes of astrocytes, but it is also present in many other tissues including kidneys, muscle and even placenta.[81–83]

There are a few important differences in pregnancy between women with NMOSD and MS. Like MS, women with NMOSD appear to be at higher risk for relapses in the first 3 months postpartum; however, unlike MS, these women are also at risk for relapse during pregnancy. These observations have been reported in several case series.[84–88] Furthermore, women with NMOSD may also experience higher rates of other pregnancy complications, such as miscarriage and preeclampsia. In one study of 40 AQP4-seropositive women with 85 pregnancies, 11 pregnancies (12.9%) ended in miscarriages: 7 were in the first trimester, 1 in the second trimester, and 3 at an unknown time within the first 24 weeks.[87] Further, rates of preeclampsia were higher among patients with NMOSD compared with the general population (11.5% vs 3.2%, respectively).[87] Finally, the mean annualized relapse rate from 9 months preconception to the end of pregnancy was higher in the miscarriage subgroup compared with the viable pregnancy subgroup.[87] This suggests that patients with more active disease may have more complications; however, further studies are needed to confirm this.

The exact immunologic mechanisms for these complications in NMOSD are unknown, but various effects of pregnancy on the AQP4-IgG antibody have been postulated.[89] Placental expression of AQP4, leading to an AQP4-antibody mediated attack on the placenta, also could be a contributing factor.[90]

There are several therapeutic options used for relapse prevention in NMOSD, including azathioprine, mycophenolate, and rituximab.[91] Rituximab has been shown in a retrospective multicenter case series of 25 patients with NMOSD to reduce the frequency of relapses, and ultimately offer stabilization or improvement in disability.[92] There are no large clinical trials of rituximab use in pregnancy, but in one case report, treatment with rituximab 1 week before unplanned pregnancy was associated with

NMO disease stability during pregnancy and no adverse events to mother and child.[93] Low B cells in newborns of mothers treated with rituximab before and during pregnancy have been reported, and appear to normalize by 6 months[94] Given the half-life of rituximab, it would theoretically be safe to begin conception attempts 3.5 to 4.0 months after infusion, after the drug has cleared maternal circulation, but still potentially offering some protection against relapses during the pregnancy. The possible risks and benefits should be weighed with each individual patient according to the patient's risk tolerance and overall disease course.

SUMMARY

Women of childbearing age with MS or NMOSD should be asked about reproductive plans at every visit. In general, women with MS should not be discouraged from pregnancy due to their illness; however, it is important to provide a framework to discuss DMT safety in pregnancy and breastfeeding, as well as uncertainty about the course of their disease during pregnancy, postpartum, and long-term.[95]

Women with NMOSD may not experience the same relatively benign course during pregnancy as patients with MS. Specific recommendations regarding whether and when to discontinue DMTs will likely continue to evolve.

Providers and patients should have open discussions about selecting appropriate DMTs, considering how to optimize chances of conceiving off DMT, reducing risks to the fetus, and ensuring a benign postpartum period.

REFERENCES

1. Bove R, Chitnis T. The role of gender and sex hormones in determining the onset and outcome of multiple sclerosis. Mult Scler 2014;20(5):520–6.
2. Douglass LH, Jorgensen CL. Pregnancy and multiple sclerosis. Am J Obstet Gynecol 1948;55:332–6.
3. Confavreux C, Hutchinson M, Hours MM, et al. Rate of pregnancy-related relapse in multiple sclerosis. N Engl J Med 1998;339(5):285–91.
4. Vukusic S, Hutchinson M, Hours M, et al. Pregnancy and multiple sclerosis (the PRIMS study): clinical predictors of post-partum relapse. Brain 2004;127(6): 1353–60.
5. Marrie RA, Gryba C. The incidence and prevalence of neuromyelitis optica: a systematic review. Int J MS Care 2013;15(3):113–8.
6. Mealy MA, Wingerchuk DM, Greenberg BM, et al. Epidemiology of neuromyelitis optica in the United States: a multicenter analysis. Arch Neurol 2012;69(9): 1176–80.
7. Wingerchuk DM, Lennon VA, Lucchinetti CF, et al. The spectrum of neuromyelitis optica. Lancet Neurol 2007;6(9):805–15.
8. Salemi G, Callari G, Gammino M, et al. The relapse rate of multiple sclerosis changes during pregnancy: a cohort study. Acta Neurol Scand 2004;110(1): 23–6.
9. Hanulíková P, Vlk R, Meluzínová E, et al. Pregnancy and multiple sclerosis—outcomes analysis 2003-2011. Ceska Gynekol 2013;78(2):142–8 [in Czech].
10. Stenager E, Stenager E, Jensen K. Effect of pregnancy on the prognosis for multiple sclerosis. A 5-year follow up investigation. Acta Neurol Scand 1994;90(5): 305–8.
11. Mueller BA, Zhang J, Critchlow CW. Birth outcomes and need for hospitalization after delivery among women with multiple sclerosis. Am J Obstet Gynecol 2002; 186(3):446–52.

12. Hellwig K, Correale J. Artificial reproductive techniques in multiple sclerosis. Clin Immunol 2013;149(2):219–24.
13. Thöne J, Kollar S, Nousome D, et al. Serum anti-Müllerian hormone levels in reproductive-age women with relapsing–remitting multiple sclerosis. Mult Scler 2015;21(1):41–7.
14. Grinsted L, Heltberg A, Hagen C, et al. Serum sex hormone and gonadotropin concentrations in premenopausal women with multiple sclerosis. J Intern Med 1989;226(4):241–4.
15. Cavalla P, Rovei V, Masera S, et al. Fertility in patients with multiple sclerosis: current knowledge and future perspectives. Neurol Sci 2006;27(4):231–9.
16. Bove R, Alwan S, Friedman JM, et al. Management of multiple sclerosis during pregnancy and the reproductive years: a systematic review. Obstet Gynecol 2014;124(6):1157–68.
17. Ascherio A, Munger KL, Lünemann JD. The initiation and prevention of multiple sclerosis. Nat Rev Neurol 2012;8(11):602–12.
18. Munger KL, Åivo J, Hongell K, et al. Vitamin D status during pregnancy and risk of multiple sclerosis in offspring of women in the Finnish maternity cohort. JAMA Neurol 2016;73(5):515–9.
19. ACOG Committee on Obstetric Practice. ACOG Committee opinion no. 495: vitamin D: screening and supplementation during pregnancy. Obstet Gynecol 2011;118:197–8.
20. Laplaud D-A, Leray E, Barriere P, et al. Increase in multiple sclerosis relapse rate following in vitro fertilization. Neurology 2006;66(8):1280–1.
21. Michel L, Foucher Y, Vukusic S, et al. Increased risk of multiple sclerosis relapse after in vitro fertilisation. J Neurol Neurosurg Psychiatry 2012;83(8):796–802.
22. Correale J, Farez MF, Ysrraelit MC. Increase in multiple sclerosis activity after assisted reproduction technology. Ann Neurol 2012;72(5):682–94.
23. Hellwig K, Beste C, Brune N, et al. Increased MS relapse rate during assisted reproduction technique. J Neurol 2008;255(4):592–3.
24. Hellwig K, Schimrigk S, Beste C, et al. Increase in relapse rate during assisted reproduction technique in patients with multiple sclerosis. Eur Neurol 2009; 61(2):65–8.
25. Bove R, Rankin K, Lin C, et al. Assisted reproductive technologies and relapse risk: a new case series, and pooled analysis of existing studies. Poster presented at ECTRIMS 2017. Paris, France, October 25–28, 2017.
26. Bove RM, Klein JP. Neuroradiology in women of childbearing age. Continuum (Minneap Minn) 2014;20(1, Neurology of Pregnancy):23–41.
27. Argyriou AA, Makris N. Multiple sclerosis and reproductive risks in women. Reprod Sci 2008;15(8):755–64.
28. Fraser F, Sajoo A. Teratogenic potential of corticosteroids in humans. Teratology 1995;51(1):45–6.
29. Carmichael SL, Shaw GM. Maternal corticosteroid use and risk of selected congenital anomalies. Am J Med Genet A 1999;86(3):242–4.
30. Skuladottir H, Wilcox AJ, Ma C, et al. Corticosteroid use and risk of orofacial clefts. Birth Defects Res A Clin Mol Teratol 2014;100(6):499–506.
31. Bay Bjørn AM, Ehrenstein V, Hundborg HH, et al. Use of corticosteroids in early pregnancy is not associated with risk of oral clefts and other congenital malformations in offspring. Am J Ther 2014;21(2):73–80.
32. Achiron A, Kishner I, Dolev M, et al. Effect of intravenous immunoglobulin treatment on pregnancy and postpartum-related relapses in multiple sclerosis. J Neurol 2004;251(9):1133–7.

33. Wundes A, Pebdani RN, Amtmann D. What do healthcare providers advise women with multiple sclerosis regarding pregnancy? Mult Scler Int 2014;2014: 819216.
34. Coyle PK. Management of women with multiple sclerosis through pregnancy and after childbirth. Ther Adv Neurol Disord 2016;9(3):198–210.
35. Amato M, Portaccio E, Ghezzi A, et al. Pregnancy and fetal outcomes after interferon-β exposure in multiple sclerosis. Neurology 2010;75(20):1794–802.
36. Boskovic R, Wide R, Wolpin J, et al. The reproductive effects of beta interferon therapy in pregnancy A longitudinal cohort. Neurology 2005;65(6):807–11.
37. Patti F, Cavallaro T, Fermo SL, et al. Is in utero early-exposure to interferon beta a risk factor for pregnancy outcomes in multiple sclerosis? J Neurol 2008;255(8): 1250–3.
38. Thiel S, Langer-Gould A, Rockhoff M, et al. Interferon-beta exposure during first trimester is safe in women with multiple sclerosis—a prospective cohort study from the German Multiple Sclerosis and Pregnancy Registry. Mult Scler 2016; 22(6):801–9.
39. Coyle PK, Sinclair S, Scheuerle A, et al. Final results from the Betaseron (interferon β-1b) Pregnancy Registry: a prospective observational study of birth defects and pregnancy-related adverse events. BMJ Open 2014;4(5):e004536.
40. Lu E, Wang BW, Guimond C, et al. Disease-modifying drugs for multiple sclerosis in pregnancy: a systematic review. Neurology 2012;79(11):1130–5.
41. Waubant E, Sadovnick AD. Interferon beta babies. Neurology 2005;65(6):788–9.
42. Fragoso YD, Finkelsztejn A, Kaimen-Maciel DR, et al. Long-term use of glatiramer acetate by 11 pregnant women with multiple sclerosis. CNS Drugs 2010;24(11): 969–76.
43. Herbstritt S, Langer-Gould A, Rockhoff M, et al. Glatiramer acetate during early pregnancy: a prospective cohort study. Mult Scler 2016;22(6):810–6.
44. Neudorfer O, Melamed-Gal S, Baruch P. Pregnancy outcomes in patients with multiple sclerosis and exposure to branded glatiramer acetate during all three trimesters. Poster presented at ECTRIMS 2017. Paris, France, October 25–28, 2017.
45. Gold R, Phillips JT, Havrdova E, et al. Delayed-release dimethyl fumarate and pregnancy: preclinical studies and pregnancy outcomes from clinical trials and postmarketing experience. Neurol Ther 2015;4(2):93–104.
46. Tecfidera, dimethy; fumarte [package insert] Cambridge,. MA: Biogen Idec; 2014.
47. Karlsson G, Francis G, Koren G, et al. Pregnancy outcomes in the clinical development program of fingolimod in multiple sclerosis. Neurology 2014;82(8): 674–80.
48. Houtchens MK, Sadovnick AD. Health issues in women with multiple sclerosis. Springer; 2017.
49. Collins W, Francis G, Koren G, et al. Lack of interaction between fingolimod (FTY720) and oral contraceptives, and pregnancy experience in the clinical program of fingolimod in multiple sclerosis. Paper presented at: Neurology2011.
50. Buraga I, Popovici R-E. Multiple sclerosis and pregnancy: current considerations. ScientificWorldJournal 2014;2014:513160.
51. Hatcher SE, Waubant E, Nourbakhsh B, et al. Rebound syndrome in patients with multiple sclerosis after cessation of fingolimod treatment. JAMA Neurol 2016; 73(7):790–4.
52. Vukusic S, Marignier R. Multiple sclerosis and pregnancy in the 'treatment era. Nat Rev Neurol 2015;11(5):280–9.

53. Brent Robert L. Teratogen update—reproductive risks of leflunomide (Arava TM); a pyrimidine synthesis inhibitor: counseling women taking leflunomide before or during pregnancy and men taking leflunomide who are contemplating fathering a child. Teratology 2001;63:106–12.

54. Cassina M, Johnson D, Robinson L, et al. Pregnancy outcome in women exposed to leflunomide before or during pregnancy. Arthritis Rheumatol 2012;64(7): 2085–94.

55. AUBAGIO prescribing information. Cambridge (England): Genzyme Corporation, a Sanofi company; 2012. Available at: http://products.sanofi.us/aubagio/aubagio. pdf. Accessed January 18, 2018.

56. Haghikia A, Langer-Gould A, Rellensmann G, et al. Natalizumab use during the third trimester of pregnancy. JAMA Neurol 2014;71(7):891–5.

57. Kümpfel T, Thiel S, Meinl I, et al. Long-term exposure to natalizumab during pregnancy—a prospective case series from the German Multiple Sclerosis and Pregnancy Registry. Poster presented at ECTRIMS 2017. Paris, France, Oct 25–28, 2017.

58. Gelfand JM, Cree BA, Hauser SL. Ocrelizumab and other CD20+ B-cell-depleting therapies in multiple sclerosis. Neurotherapeutics 2017;14(4):835–41.

59. Klink D, Van Elburg R, Schreurs M, et al. Rituximab administration in third trimester of pregnancy suppresses neonatal B-cell development. Clin Dev Immunol 2008;2008(1):1.

60. Chakravarty EF, Murray ER, Kelman A, et al. Pregnancy outcomes after maternal exposure to rituximab. Blood 2011;117(5):1499–506.

61. Ocrelizumab [package insert]. San Francisco (CA): Genentech; 2017.

62. Oh J, Achiron A, Chambers C, et al. Pregnancy outcomes in patients with RRMS who received alemtuzumab in the clinical development program (S24. 008). Neurology 2016;86(16 Supplement):S24–2008.

63. Thöne J, Thiel S, Gold R, et al. Treatment of multiple sclerosis during pregnancy–safety considerations. Expert Opin Drug Saf 2017;16(5):523–34.

64. Langer-Gould A, Beaber BE. Effects of pregnancy and breastfeeding on the multiple sclerosis disease course. Clin Immunol 2013;149(2):244–50.

65. Hellwig K, Rockhoff M, Herbstritt S, et al. Exclusive breastfeeding and the effect on postpartum multiple sclerosis relapses. JAMA Neurol 2015;72(10):1132–8.

66. Portaccio E, Ghezzi A, Hakiki B, et al. Breastfeeding is not related to postpartum relapses in multiple sclerosis. Neurology 2011;77(2):145–50.

67. Pakpoor J, Disanto G, Lacey MV, et al. Breastfeeding and multiple sclerosis relapses: a meta-analysis. J Neurol 2012;259(10):2246–8.

68. Hale TW, Siddiqui AA, Baker TE. Transfer of interferon β-1a into human breastmilk. Breastfeed Med 2012;7(2):123–5.

69. Voskuhl R, Momtazee C. Pregnancy: effect on multiple sclerosis, treatment considerations, and breastfeeding. Neurotherapeutics 2017;14(4):974–84.

70. Hellwig K. Pregnancy in multiple sclerosis. Eur Neurol 2014;72(Suppl. 1):39–42.

71. Almas S, Vance J, Baker T, et al. Management of multiple sclerosis in the breastfeeding mother. Mult Scler Int 2016;2016:6527458.

72. Baker TE, Cooper SD, Kessler L, et al. Transfer of natalizumab into breast milk in a mother with multiple sclerosis. J Hum Lact 2015;31(2):233–6.

73. Vaidyanathan A, McKeever K, Anand B, et al. Developmental immunotoxicology assessment of rituximab in cynomolgus monkeys. Toxicol Sci 2010;119(1): 116–25.

74. Hurley WL, Theil PK. Perspectives on immunoglobulins in colostrum and milk. Nutrients 2011;3(4):442–74.

75. Bragnes Y, Boshuizen R, de Vries A, et al. Low level of rituximab in human breast milk in a patient treated during lactation. Rheumatology 2017;56(6):1047–8.
76. De Seze J, Chapelotte M, Delalande S, et al. Intravenous corticosteroids in the postpartum period for reduction of acute exacerbations in multiple sclerosis. Mult Scler 2004;10(5):596–7.
77. Cooper SD, Felkins K, Baker TE, et al. Transfer of methylprednisolone into breast milk in a mother with multiple sclerosis. J Hum Lact 2015;31(2):237–9.
78. Achiron A, Rotstein Z, Noy S, et al. Intravenous immunoglobulin treatment in the prevention of childbirth-associated acute exacerbations in multiple sclerosis: a pilot study. J Neurol 1996;243(1):25–8.
79. Brandt-Wouters E, Gerlach OH, Hupperts RM. The effect of postpartum intravenous immunoglobulins on the relapse rate among patients with multiple sclerosis. Int J Gynaecol Obstet 2016;134(2):194–6.
80. Pandit L, Asgari N, Apiwattanakul M, et al. Demographic and clinical features of neuromyelitis optica: a review. Mult Scler 2015;21(7):845–53.
81. Quek AM, McKeon A, Lennon VA, et al. Effects of age and sex on aquaporin-4 autoimmunity. Arch Neurol 2012;69(8):1039–43.
82. Lennon VA, Kryzer TJ, Pittock SJ, et al. IgG marker of optic-spinal multiple sclerosis binds to the aquaporin-4 water channel. J Exp Med 2005;202(4):473–7.
83. Matiello M, Schaefer-Klein J, Sun D, et al. Aquaporin 4 expression and tissue susceptibility to neuromyelitis optica. JAMA Neurol 2013;70(9):1118–25.
84. Klawiter EC, Bove R, Elsone L, et al. High risk of postpartum relapses in neuromyelitis optica spectrum disorder. Neurology 2017. https://doi.org/10.1212/WNL. 0000000000004681.
85. Kim W, Kim S-H, Nakashima I, et al. Influence of pregnancy on neuromyelitis optica spectrum disorder. Neurology 2012;78(16):1264–7.
86. Fragoso YD, Adoni T, Bichuetti DB, et al. Neuromyelitis optica and pregnancy. J Neurol 2013;260(10):2614–9.
87. Nour MM, Nakashima I, Coutinho E, et al. Pregnancy outcomes in aquaporin-4–positive neuromyelitis optica spectrum disorder. Neurology 2016;86(1):79–87.
88. Reichlin M. Systemic lupus erythematosus and pregnancy. J Reprod Med 1998;43:355–60.
89. Davoudi V, Keyhanian K, Bove RM, et al. Immunology of neuromyelitis optica during pregnancy. Neurol Neuroimmunol Neuroinflamm 2016;3(6):e288.
90. Reuß R, Rommer PS, Brück W, et al. A woman with acute myelopathy in pregnancy: case outcome. United Kingdom: BMJ Publishing Group; 2009.
91. Kimbrough DJ, Fujihara K, Jacob A, et al. Treatment of neuromyelitis optica: review and recommendations. Mult Scler Relat Disord 2012;1(4):180–7.
92. Jacob A, Weinshenker BG, Violich I, et al. Treatment of neuromyelitis optica with rituximab. Arch Neurol 2008;65(11):1443–8.
93. Pellkofer H, Suessmair C, Schulze A, et al. Course of neuromyelitis optica during inadvertent pregnancy in a patient treated with rituximab. Mult Scler 2009;15(8):1006–8.
94. Azim HA Jr, Azim H, Peccatori FA. Treatment of cancer during pregnancy with monoclonal antibodies: a real challenge. Expert Rev Clin Immunol 2010;6(6):821–6.
95. Prunty M, Sharpe L, Butow P, et al. The motherhood choice: themes arising in the decision-making process for women with multiple sclerosis. Mult Scler 2008;14(5):701–4.

Headache in Pregnancy and the Puerperium

Rebecca Burch, MD

KEYWORDS

- Headache • Migraine • Migraine with aura • Pregnancy • Postpartum • Lactation
- Treatment

KEY POINTS

- Migraine is the most common cause of headache during pregnancy. Migraine improves after the first trimester in approximately two-thirds of women but may persist. Migraine, especially migraine with aura, may present for the first time during pregnancy.
- Important causes of secondary headache include vascular disorders, such as preeclampsia, reversible cerebral vasoconstriction syndrome, and cerebral venous thrombosis, as well as idiopathic intracranial hypertension.
- In addition to recurrent or incident migraine, postdural puncture headache is a common cause of headache during the postpartum period. Early blood patch may be warranted if the headache is disabling.
- Nonpharmacologic treatments of migraine are emphasized during pregnancy. There is growing evidence supporting the use of triptans rather than butalbital combination analgesics as second-line treatments after acetaminophen. Propranolol is the preferred preventive treatment, and amitriptyline and verapamil are second line.
- Treatment of migraine during lactation is typically less restrictive than during pregnancy.

INTRODUCTION

Migraine or severe headache disorders are reported by approximately 20% of women in the United States at any given time.[1] Migraine and severe headache are more common in women and are most active in women of reproductive age.[2] Migraine is a frequent cause of headache during pregnancy and the postpartum period (puerperium), but pregnancy and the first 6 weeks after delivery are also associated with an increased risk for many concerning causes of headache. This review focuses on diagnosis and work-up of different headaches types that may present during pregnancy and the immediate postpartum period. Management of migraine during pregnancy and during lactation also are discussed.

Conflicts of Interest Statement: The author has no relevant conflicts of interest to disclose.
Department of Neurology, John R. Graham Headache Center, Brigham and Women's Hospital, Harvard Medical School, 1153 Centre Street, Suite 4H, Jamaica Plain, Boston, MA 02130, USA
E-mail address: rburch@partners.org

Neurol Clin 37 (2019) 31–51
https://doi.org/10.1016/j.ncl.2018.09.004
0733-8619/19/© 2018 Elsevier Inc. All rights reserved.

neurologic.theclinics.com

APPROACH TO THE PREGNANT OR POSTPARTUM PATIENT WITH HEADACHE

The International Classification of Headache Disorders (ICHD) divides headaches into primary and secondary categories.[3] Primary headaches, including migraine and tension-type headache, do not have a clear underlying causative pathology and are diagnosed according to their phenomenology. Secondary headaches are caused by an identifiable abnormality, and the list of etiologies for secondary headaches is extensive. A large majority of the secondary headaches seen in pregnancy and the puerperium are caused by vascular disorders, in particular conditions associated with gestational hypertension.[4,5] Disorders of high or low cerebrospinal fluid (CSF) pressure, including postdural puncture headache, are also a significant cause of secondary headache, particularly in the postpartum period. Selected concerning clinical scenarios and potential causes are listed in **Table 1**.

Table 1
Concerning presentations of headache

Presentation	Possible Etiology	Work-up
Thunderclap headache	Subarachnoid or intraparenchymal hemorrhage Ischemic stroke RCVS Preeclampsia/eclampsia CVT PRES Pituitary apoplexy Arterial dissection	• Consider CT/LP to rule out hemorrhage • MRI/MRA/MRV, consider including neck MRA • Assess for proteinuria, hypertension • Consider repeat MRA in 2–4 wk if suspicion of RCVS is high
Chronic, progressive, refractory headache	CVT Migraine Tumor, including microadenoma	• MRI/MRV
Headache associated with visual symptoms	Migraine aura Ischemic stroke Preeclampsia IIH	• Fundoscopic examination • MRI/MRV • Assess for proteinuria, hypertension • Lumbar puncture for manometry • Visual field testing
Headache associated with neurologic signs or symptoms	Ischemic or hemorrhagic stroke CVT PRES Preeclampsia Arterial dissection Migraine aura	• MRI/MRA/MRV, consider including neck MRA • Assess for proteinuria, hypertension
Headache associated with proteinuria, hypertension, or seizure	Preeclampsia/eclampsia PRES	• MRI/MRA to rule out overlapping vascular pathologies, such as RCVS
Headache worsening with Valsalva Maneuver, straining, heavy lifting; papilledema	CVT IIH Tumor	• MRI/MRV • Lumbar puncture for manometry • Visual field testing
Postural headache in the postpartum period	Postdural puncture headache	• MRI • Empiric blood patch

Abbreviations: CT, Computed Tomography; LP, Lumbar Puncture; MRA, Magnetic Resonance Angiography; MRV, Magnetic Resonance Venography; PRES, Posterior reversible encephalopathy syndrome.

Migraine and tension-type headaches are the most common cause of headaches during pregnancy.[6] Red flags in the clinical history or on neurologic examination, summarized in **Box 1**, should raise concern for an underlying secondary headache. It is important to remember that women with a history of migraine also may present with secondary headaches. Migraine, in particular migraine with aura, is a risk factor for preeclampsia, cerebral venous thrombosis (CVT), and stroke during pregnancy.[7] A headache that a patient reports as qualitatively different from her usual symptoms should raise concern for another, potentially serious, cause. Observational studies of patients requiring neurologic consultation for headache during pregnancy found that absence of prior headache history and presence of hypertension, fever, and abnormal neurologic findings were the factors most predictive of secondary headache.[4,5]

In the puerperium, up to 40% of women experience headache within the first several weeks.[8] A majority of these headaches are caused by primary headache disorders, but the vascular processes active in pregnancy also can cause postpartum headache. The risk of preeclampsia or other vascular conditions does not resolve immediately after delivery, and, for some conditions, such as reversible cerebral vasoconstriction syndrome (RCVS) and CVT, risk may actually increase. In 1 study describing diagnoses made after neurologic consultation for postpartum headache, a majority were secondary headaches.[9] Of these, postdural puncture headache was the most common, followed by postpartum preeclampsia and then other vascular disorders. This study suggests that secondary causes should strongly be considered when a woman presents with bothersome headaches during the puerperium.

Imaging of the brain and blood vessels is necessary in almost all cases of secondary headache strongly suspected. There are few good studies regarding safety of either brain MRI or head CT in pregnant women. MRI is preferable to CT due to the radiation exposure associated with CT.[10] Despite this, the fetal radiation exposure from a maternal CT scan of the head is very low, and CT can be considered if clinically necessary. Gadolinium should be avoided unless absolutely necessary because animal studies have shown embryocidal effects at high doses.[10]

DIFFERENTIAL DIAGNOSIS OF HEADACHE DURING AND AFTER PREGNANCY
Migraine

21% to 28% of women are estimated to experience migraine between the ages of 18 to 49, and 80% of women with migraine continue to experience attacks during some

---

Box 1
Red flags in clinical history or neurologic examination

Clinical signs
  Sudden onset (thunderclap headache)
  Progressive, worsening
  Change from prior headache type
  Refractory to treatment
  Worsening with Valsalva Maneuver, straining, coughing, or sneezing
  Worsens with posture (sitting or standing)

Examination or laboratory findings
  Papilledema
  Peripheral edema
  Hypertension
  Focal neurologic findings (numbness, weakness)
  Fever
  Seizure

portion of pregnancy.[2,11] Approximately two-thirds of woman experience improvement in their migraines during the second and third trimesters.[6] Women with migraine with aura, however, may be less likely to experience improvement. Migraine is characterized by a headache lasting between 4 hours and 72 hours, with at least 2 of the 4 following pain characteristics: unilateral, pulsating or throbbing in quality, moderate to severe, and worsening with or causing avoidance of physical activity. It must be accompanied by either nausea or vomiting or both photophobia and phonophobia. The ICHD requires 5 attacks before a diagnosis of primary migraine headache can be made.[3] Despite this, some women present with migraine for the first time during pregnancy.

The initial presentation of migraine aura may also occur during pregnancy, either in women with no history of migraine or with a history of migraine without aura.[12] Elevated estrogen levels and/or the lack of estrogen cycling associated with pregnancy are believed to reduce the threshold for cortical spreading depression, the pathophysiologic cause of aura. The diagnostic criteria for migraine aura are found in **Box 2**. Migraine aura should be differentiated from cerebral infarction, the visual symptoms related to preeclampsia, and the transient visual obscurations associated with elevated intracranial pressure. The presence of positive rather than negative symptoms supports a diagnosis of migraine aura, as does a discrete time course and a temporal relationship to headache.[13]

Primary headaches, including migraine and tension-type headaches, are also the most common headaches occurring during the puerperium.[8] Physiologic changes, such as falling estrogen levels and changes in endothelial function, contribute to migraine susceptibility along with environmental factors, such as disrupted sleep and increased stress. One prospective study showed that 34% of women had recurrence of migraine within the first week after delivery and 55% had recurrence within the first month.[14] Another study found that 5% of women presented with their first-ever migraine in the postpartum period.[15]

Preeclampsia/Eclampsia, Reversible Cerebral Vasoconstriction Syndrome, and Posterior Reversible Encephalopathy Syndrome

These conditions, preeclampsia/eclampsia, RCVS, and posterior reversible encephalopathy syndrome, although diagnosed separately, have significant clinical and pathophysiologic overlap. They are characterized by endothelial dysfunction and increased vascular tone. These processes leads to a constellation of symptoms, including systemic hypertension, cerebral vasospasm, cerebral edema, and other systemic end organ damage. The pathophysiology of these diseases is discussed in more detail in another article included in this issue.

Box 2
International Classification of Headache Disorders criteria for migraine aura

1. Aura symptoms may be visual, sensory, speech and/or language, motor, brainstem, retinal

2. Symptoms should have at least 3 of the following characteristics:
   - At least 1 aura symptom spreads gradually over ≥5 minutes
   - Two or more aura symptoms occur in succession
   - Each individual aura symptom lasts 5 minutes to 60 minutes
   - At least 1 aura symptom is unilateral
   - At least 1 aura symptom is positive
   - The aura is accompanied, or followed within 60 minutes, by headache

Preeclampsia is defined as gestational hypertension (systolic blood pressure over 140 mm Hg or diastolic blood pressure over 90 mm Hg) associated with symptoms of end organ damage.[16] Proteinuria can be 1 such symptom but is no longer required for diagnosis per American College of Obstetricians and Gynecologists criteria revised in 2013. Thrombocytopenia, renal insufficiency, impaired liver function, pulmonary edema, and cerebral or visual symptoms, including headache, are other qualifying symptoms. Per the revised criteria, headache in the presence of gestational hypertension is sufficient to make a diagnosis of preeclampsia.

The headache is most often progressive and does not respond well to treatment. Visual symptoms, including scotoma and blurry vision, may accompany preeclampsia and can be mistaken for migraine aura. Historically it has been believed that the progressive, refractory nature of the headache could differentiate preeclampsia from migraine. A recent study found that there were no clinically meaningful features differentiating the 2 headaches, however.[9] A work-up for preeclampsia in any pregnant or postpartum woman with new or different headache should be considered.

Eclampsia is defined as a seizure in a patient with preeclampsia, but eclamptic seizures may also occur in women who did not have previously diagnosed hypertension or proteinuria.[17] Eclampsia develops in approximately 2% of women with preeclampsia. At least half of women experience a headache prior to the first eclamptic seizure.[17]

Recurrent thunderclap headache is the most common presentation of RCVS.[18] Thunderclap headache is an acute-onset headache that is maximal within a few seconds and often has an explosive quality. RCVS is characterized by segmental cerebral vasoconstriction that spontaneously reverses on imaging within 3 months. The vasospasm starts at the periphery and progresses toward the larger, more central blood vessels. For this reason, vascular imaging can be negative at the time of headache onset, and imaging may be repeated in 2 weeks to 4 weeks if there is high suspicion and results are used to guide treatment.[19] RCVS can be associated with hemorrhagic and ischemic stroke. RCVS also may occur in concert with preeclampsia or eclampsia or may be isolated. In addition to pregnancy, risk factors for RCVS include exposure to serotonergic or vasoconstricting substances, such as selective serotonin reuptake inhibitors/selective norepinephrine reuptake inhibitors, triptans, pseudoephedrine, and cocaine. Marijuana use also has been linked to increased risk. RCVS is more common in the puerperium than during pregnancy and has been historically known as postpartum angiopathy in this setting.

Cerebral Venous Thrombosis

Pregnancy is also a risk factor for systemic venous thrombosis, including CVT, because elevated estrogen levels during pregnancy have a prothombotic effect. It is more common in women with an underlying hypercoagulable disorder, and CVT during the first trimester may be the first presentation.[20] CVT presents as thunderclap headache approximately 10% of the time but more typically is associated with a slower onset, chronic, unremitting headache accompanied by symptoms of increased intracranial pressure.[21] Headache may be absent in another 10% of patients.[22] With progression of the thrombosis, neurologic deficits ranging from focal findings to coma also can occur. The focality of neurologic findings does not typically follow a known arterial pattern and can be missed more easily than arterial cerebral infarction. Seizures can also occur in patients with CVT.

Three-quarters of pregnancy-associated cases of CVT occur in the puerperium.[23] It is more common in women who had a traumatic delivery or caesarean section, postdural puncture CSF leak, dehydration, or anemia as well as those with hypercoagulable disorders.

Idiopathic Intracranial Hypertension

Studies are conflicting as to whether pregnancy is a risk factor for idiopathic intracranial hypertension (IIH).[24] The current balance of evidence suggests that although IIH may occur during pregnancy, pregnancy itself does not increase the likelihood of developing IIH. IIH may also occur for the first time in the postpartum period.[25] The diagnosis should be suspected in a patient with headaches that worsen with exertion, straining, Valsalva Maneuver, or lying down. A majority of patients report transient visual obscurations, particularly with exertional maneuvers, and pulsatile tinnitus is present in half of patients.[26] Fundoscopic examination almost always shows papilledema, but rare cases of elevated intracranial pressure without papilledema have been reported. MRI of the brain should be performed to rule out a space-occupying lesion. Lumbar puncture showing an opening pressure of at least 25 cm of water is required for the diagnosis. Visual field testing should be done to document the extent of any visual loss and track response to treatment. The treatment of choice in a nonpregnant patient is acetazolamide.[26] Historically there have been concerns about use of acetazolamide during pregnancy due to evidence of fetal toxicity in animal studies. Recent studies have not shown an increased risk of congenital malformation with acetazolamide use.[27] IIH during pregnancy can also be managed with serial lumbar punctures.

Postdural Puncture Headache

Postpartum headache due to CSF leak and subsequent low intracranial pressure is most often secondary to dural puncture. This known complication of epidural anesthesia occurs in approximately 1% of cases.[28] Young women with a low body mass index are at higher risk. Although rare, a CSF leak can also develop without dural puncture and may be related to straining during the second stage of labor. The hallmark of low CSF pressure headache is improvement of pain when lying supine and recurrence of headache when the patient is upright.[3] Some patients improve with rest, intravenous (IV) fluids, and possibly caffeine. Epidural blood patch should be performed if the headache is severe and limiting or if no improvement of milder headache is seen after several days. Inability to sit or stand can be highly disabling for new mothers and early treatment with a blood patch should be strongly considered. Up to a third of patients who receive a blood patch need repeat treatment.[29]

Other

Other less common but potentially dangerous causes of headache during pregnancy and the puerperium include subarachnoid or intraparenchymal hemorrhage, pituitary adenoma or apoplexy, arterial dissection, acute cerebral infarction, and infection.[4] Women with a history of migraine may be at higher risk for carotid artery dissection.[30] Strain related to pushing during the second stage of labor may also increase risk of arterial dissection.

MANAGEMENT OF MIGRAINE DURING PREGNANCY

Women with severe or frequent migraines may be apprehensive about treatment limitations during pregnancy. Women considering pregnancy or during early pregnancy should be reassured that there are many treatment options available, that their providers will work with them to manage their headaches, and that migraines often (although not always) improve after the first trimester.[6]

Treatment of migraine during pregnancy emphasizes lifestyle management and nonpharmacologic approaches. Biofeedback and relaxation practices have good evidence for efficacy as preventive treatments and may be effective for aborting migraine in the early stages.[31] These techniques are most effective when practiced regularly and should ideally be started prior to pregnancy. Adequate and good-quality sleep, regular meals, hydration, and maintaining an exercise program are positive lifestyle features that can reduce frequency of migraine and can also be initiated prior to pregnancy.

A preconception visit can also include education about the menstrual cycle. If a woman has regular menstrual cycles, she may be able to predict ovulation and menstruation times. Between menstruation and ovulation, there are no restrictions on acute medication use. Shortening the window during which medications must be restricted can reduce migraine-related disability during attempts to conceive.

Information regarding medication safety during pregnancy is limited. Few medications are tested for safety in pregnant women, and the majority of information regarding medication safety in pregnancy is based on observational or registry studies. In 2014, the US Food and Drug Administration (FDA) retired the letter categorization system describing risk associated with medication use in pregnancy (**Box 3**).[32] There is currently no formal grading system for medication safety, and clinicians are instead expected to rely on their interpretation of the available evidence. Many clinicians still find it useful to consider the former FDA risk in pregnancy letter grade. In this article, both the FDA pregnancy risk letter categories (referred to as pregnancy category) and a brief summary of available evidence are described.

Despite this uncertainty, withholding treatment of migraine during pregnancy is also not without risk. Migraine attacks may be associated with low caloric intake, dehydration, and electrolyte imbalances due to vomiting.[33] Frequent severe migraine may also lead to a high burden of missed work days or decreased productivity at work.[34] Pain may also be a risk factor for physical and mental health issues during pregnancy and the postpartum period.[35,36] Treatment should strongly be considered in situations where any of these negative consequences are likely.

Box 3
Food and Drug Administration pregnancy risk letter categories

A: Adequate and well-controlled studies have failed to demonstrate a risk to the fetus in the first trimester of pregnancy (and there is no evidence of risk in later trimesters).

B: Animal reproduction studies have failed to demonstrate a risk to the fetus and there are no adequate and well-controlled studies in pregnant women.

C: Animal reproduction studies have shown an adverse effect on the fetus and there are no adequate and well-controlled studies in humans, but potential benefits may warrant use of the drug in pregnant women despite potential risks.

D: There is positive evidence of human fetal risk based on adverse reaction data from investigational or marketing experience or studies in humans, but potential benefits may warrant use of the drug in pregnant women despite potential risks.

X: Studies in animals or humans have demonstrated fetal abnormalities and/or there is positive evidence of human fetal risk based on adverse reaction data from investigational or marketing experience, and the risks involved in use of the drug in pregnant women clearly outweigh potential benefits.

Acute Treatment

The safety evidence for commonly used abortive treatments in pregnancy is summarized in **Table 2**. Acetaminophen and metoclopramide are traditional first-line therapies in addition to topical ice, rest, and relaxation or biofeedback techniques. Acetaminophen was in pregnancy category B and is generally believed safe during pregnancy. Ibuprofen may be used safely during the second trimester. Use in the first trimester may increase the risk of miscarriage.[37] Exposure to nonsteroidal anti-inflammatory drugs (NSAIDs) during the third trimester may cause premature closure of the fetal ductus arteriosus and is thus contraindicated.

Butalbital combination medications have traditionally been preferred as second-line symptomatic treatment. The available evidence suggests that triptans may be equally, or more, safe during pregnancy. A 2015 meta-analysis of pregnancy outcomes after exposure to triptans included 4208 infants and found no significant increase in major congenital malformations, premature birth, or spontaneous abortions among triptan users compared with women with migraine who did not use triptans.[38] Recent American Headache Society guidelines for acute treatment of migraine found level A evidence ("established as effective") for use of triptans but only level C evidence ("possibly effective") for butalbital combination medications.[39] If treatment with a triptan is more effective, fewer doses of acute medication may be required and the overall burden of medication may be lower. Providers should strongly consider whether triptan use may be appropriate as a second-line treatment, especially in patients who are known to respond well to triptans.

Rescue therapy may be needed if a migraine attack does not respond to first-line or second-line therapies. At-home treatments might include sedative antiemetics (such as diphenhydramine) and encouraging fluids, and it may be reasonable to consider rare use of an opiate in this case. In urgent care or emergency room settings, IV fluids, metoclopramide, diphenhydramine, and an NSAID (during the second trimester) can be used. Parenteral opioids should be avoided, as is the case outside of pregnancy. A recent study comparing IV metoclopramide and diphenhydramine to oral codeine in women who had failed acetaminophen therapy found that these treatments were equally effective.[40] Occipital nerve blocks using lidocaine alone are helpful in the office setting and are considered compatible with pregnancy. Ergots, including dihydroergotamine, which cause vasoconstriction and increase the risk of pregnancy loss, should be avoided at all times during pregnancy.

Preventive Treatment

The safety evidence for commonly used preventive treatments in pregnancy is summarized in **Table 3**. Prevention should be considered in women who have frequent, moderate to severe attacks that do not respond well to acute treatment.[33] Propranolol is the preventive with the best evidence for safe use during pregnancy and is preferred as the first-line preventive treatment. Amitriptyline and verapamil have a lower risk profile than other preventive options and are second-line preventive treatments. Most antiepileptics, including topiramate and valproate, are contraindicated due to known teratogenic risks. Onabotulinum toxin A is currently not recommended for use during pregnancy. Although it is unlikely that this large protein crosses the placenta, it is unknown whether there are rare uterine or placental effects that may increase the risk of fetal malformations.[41] Because onabotulinum toxin has a long duration of action, pregnancy should not be attempted until 12 weeks after the last exposure.

Many women who currently use preventive treatment of migraine wish to become pregnant. Because most women with migraine experience improvement in their

Table 2
Commonly used abortive medications for migraine and safety during pregnancy

Medication	Food and Drug Administration Pregnancy Category	Available Pregnancy Safety Information	Hale's Lactation Risk Rating	Available Lactation Safety Information
Analgesics and NSAIDS				
Acetominophen	B	No increased risk of teratogenic effects, spontaneous abortion, or stillbirth. Case reports of prenatal closure of the ductus arteriosus reported with use during the third trimester; increased risk of early childhood wheezing and asthma reported with frequent maternal use.	L1 (compatible)	Preferred. Infant exposure in breastmilk much lower than typically used therapeutic doses used for infants.
Aspirin	C	Increased risk of fetal/neonatal hemorrhage, perinatal mortality by intrauterine growth restriction, and teratogenic effects with chronic medium to high doses. In third trimester, may cause premature closure of the ductus arteriosus.	L2 (probably compatible)	Other agents strongly preferred. avoid chronic use; with occasional use, monitor infant for hemolysis, prolonged bleeding, metabolic acidosis.
NSAIDs	B (ibuprofen, naproxen, diclofenac) C (indomethacin)	Use restricted to second trimester. Use in first trimester linked to increased risk of spontaneous abortion. Use in third trimester may cause premature closure of the ductus arteriosus. Ibuprofen has the best data for safety.	L1 (compatible): ibuprofen; L2 (probably compatible): diclofenac L3 (no data—probably compatible): naproxen, indomethacin	Adverse events not reported in breastfeeding infants. Avoid in mothers of infants with platelet dysfunction or thrombocytopenia. Best evidence for ibuprofen; poor data for indomethacin.

(continued on next page)

Table 2
(continued)

Medication	Food and Drug Administration Pregnancy Category	Available Pregnancy Safety Information	Hale's Lactation Risk Rating	Available Lactation Safety Information
Butalbital	C	Long history of use in pregnancy. One large study showed possible increase in risk of fetal heart defects when butalbital used in periconceptual period; another large study showed no increase in risk. Withdrawal seizures and barbiturate withdrawal symptoms have been reported in infants after maternal use in the third trimester.	L3 (no data—probably compatible)	Concern for sedation in infant.
Opiates (oxycodone, hydromorphone, hydrocodone, codeine)	C	Either no information regarding risk of fetal malformations or no increase in risk of major congenital malformations; neonatal abstinence syndromes seen after prolonged use in later pregnancy.	L3 (no data—probably compatible): oxycodone, hydrocodone, hydromorphone; L4 (potentially hazardous): codeine	Monitor infants for respiratory depression; avoid codeine in breastfeeding mothers; codeine was associated with 1 fetal death; monitor infants exposed to codeine for sedation, apnea, bradycardia, cyanosis.
Triptans and ergots				
Triptans	C	No increased risk of major congenital malformations; studies conflicting about possible increased risk of premature birth; evidence best for sumatriptan, naratriptan, and rizatriptan.	L3 (no data—probably compatible)	No information available; eletriptan is likely to have lowest concentrations in breastmilk; avoid long-acting triptans (naratriptan and frovatriptan); option to discard pumped milk 12 h after dose if high concern.

Ergots (dihydroergotamine, ergotamine)	X	Increased risk of miscarriage.	L4 (potentially hazardous)	Avoid; may cause gastrointestinal distress and weakness in infant; may suppress milk production.
Antiemetics				
Diphenhydramine	B	No increased risk of major congenital malformations or other adverse outcomes; possible neonatal withdrawal with prolonged maternal use in third trimester.	L2 (probably compatible)	Other agents preferred; monitor for drowsiness or irritability; may reduce milk supply
Metoclopramide	B	Many studies; no increased risk of adverse pregnancy-related outcomes. May cause extrapyramidal signs and methemoglobinemia in neonates with maternal exposure during delivery.	L2 (probably compatible)	Infants may experience intestinal discomfort and gas; monitor infants for extrapyramidal symptoms and methemoglobinemia.
Promethazine	C	Other agents preferred. May cause platelet aggregation inhibition, irritability, or extrapyramidal effects in infants after maternal use within 2 wk prior to delivery.	L3 (no data—probably compatible)	Other agents preferred. May cause sedation or irritability in infants. May interfere with establishment of milk supply
Prochlorperazine	C	Other agents preferred. May cause infant jaundice, reflex changes, extrapyramidal symptoms, and potentially severe withdrawal effects after maternal use in the third trimester.	L3 (no data—probably compatible)	Effects unknown; other agents strongly preferred.

(continued on next page)

Table 2
(continued)

Medication	Food and Drug Administration Pregnancy Category	Available Pregnancy Safety Information	Hale's Lactation Risk Rating	Available Lactation Safety Information
Ondansetron	B	No increased risk of major congenital malformations, spontaneous abortion, or stillbirth; studies conflicting about possible increased risk of congenital heart malformations; the balance of evidence suggests against but study quality is challenging.	L2 (probably compatible)	No evidence.
Rescue treatments				
Prednisone	C (D for delayed-release formulations)	Increased risk of cleft lip or cleft palate, low birth weight; risks more strongly associated with chronic rather than episodic use; monitor infants for hypoadrenalism with chronic maternal use.	L2 (probably compatible)	Generally considered compatible with breastfeeding; infant exposure <0.1% of maternal dose; can pump and discard for 4 h if concern remains.
Lidocaine SQ	B	Limited data; existing studies show no increased risk of major congenital malformations; animal studies showed no teratogenic effects.	L2 (probably compatible)	Compatible with breastfeeding.

All information in this table obtained from Micromedex,[53] Natural Medicine,[53] and Reprotox[55] databases and *Hale's Medications & Mother's Milk*.

Table 3
Commonly used preventive medications for migraine and safety during pregnancy

Medication	Food and Drug Administration Pregnancy Category	Available Pregnancy Safety Information	Hale's Lactation Safety Rating	Available Lactation Safety Information
Antidepressants				
Amitriptyline	C	Second-line choice. Case reports of limb deformities, developmental delay but no causal relationship established. Monitor for infant irritability, urinary retention or constipation with late-term exposure.	L2 (probably compatible)	May be compatible. Report of infant sedation at maternal doses as low as 10 mg/d. Second line for migraine prevention; monitor infant for sedation, poor feeding.
Nortriptyline	C	Less information available than for amitriptyline; risks believed to be the same.	L2 (probably compatible)	Less information available than for amitriptyline; risks believed to be the same.
Venlafaxine	C	Other agents preferred. No increase in fetal congenital malformations; possible increased risk of spontaneous abortion; neonatal seizures, neonatal abstinence syndrome, or serotonergic toxicity possible with maternal use in third trimester.	L2 (probably compatible)	No evidence. Recommend avoidance.
Antihypertensives				
Propranolol	C	First-line choice. Observational studies show small increase in risk of intrauterine growth retardation, small placenta, and congenital abnormalities; neonatal bradycardia, respiratory depression, and hypoglycemia with late-term use	L2 (probably compatible)	Compatible with breastfeeding. Monitor infant for bradycardia, hypoglycemia.

(continued on next page)

Table 3
(continued)

Medication	Food and Drug Administration Pregnancy Category	Available Pregnancy Safety Information	Hale's Lactation Safety Rating	Available Lactation Safety Information
Verapamil	C	No increase in fetal congenital malformations; may cause fetal bradycardia, hypotension, heart block; case report of congenital cardiomyopathy after IV treatment ×2.	L2 (probably compatible)	Compatible with breastfeeding. Exposure <1% of maternal dose.
Candesartan	D	Avoid use. Risk of fetal and neonatal death with second and third trimesters exposure; may cause oligohydramnios, fetal lung hypoplasia, renal failure, skeletal deformations. May cause hypotension, oliguria, hyperkalemia in exposed infants.	L3 (no data—probably compatible)	No evidence. Recommend avoidance.
Lisinopril	D	Avoid use. Risk of fetal and neonatal death with second and third trimesters exposure; may cause oligohydramnios, fetal lung hypoplasia, renal failure, skeletal deformations. May cause hypotension, oliguria, hyperkalemia in exposed infants.	L3 (no data—probably compatible)	No evidence. Recommend avoidance.

Antiepileptics				
Topiramate	D	Avoid use. Increased risk of cleft lip or palate, small for gestational age; concern for metabolic acidosis	L3 (no data—probably compatible)	No evidence. Recommend avoidance.
Valproic acid	X	Use for migraine prophylaxis contraindicated. Increased risk of neural tube defects, craniofacial defects, cardiovascular malformations, autism, decreased IQ, and other teratogenic effects.	L4 (potentially hazardous)	Generally, compatible with breastfeeding. Monitor infant for jaundice, hepatoxicity, hematologic abnormalities.
Gabapentin	C	Limited data; no increase in fetal congenital malformations; possible increased risk of preterm birth.	L2 (probably compatible)	Possibly compatible; monitor infant for sedation, poor feeding.
Pregabalin	C	Limited data; possible increase in major congenital malformations.	L3 (no data—probably compatible)	May cause poor feeding.
Other				
Memantine	B	No data in humans; animal studies showed no teratogenic effects.	L3 (no data—probably compatible)	No evidence.
Onabotulinum Toxin A	C	Use not currently recommended; limited data; registry data do not show an increased risk of major congenital malformations.	L3 (no data—probably compatible)	No evidence; current recommendation is to avoid use.
Cyclobenzaprine	B	No data in humans; animal studies showed no teratogenic effects.	L3 (no data—probably compatible)	No evidence.
Erenumab	N/A	No data in humans; animal studies showed no teratogenic effects.	N/A	No evidence.

(continued on next page)

Table 3
(continued)

Medication	Food and Drug Administration Pregnancy Category	Available Pregnancy Safety Information	Hale's Lactation Safety Rating	Available Lactation Safety Information
Herbs and supplements				
Coenzyme Q10	N/A	Limited data; a single randomized controlled trial of CoQ10 200 mg daily in the second half of pregnancy did not show increased risk of adverse fetal outcomes.	L3 (no data—probably compatible)	No evidence; recommend avoidance.
Vitamin B₂	N/A	Safe at physiologic doses; no evidence for use at supraphysiologic doses.	L1 (compatible) at physiologic doses	No evidence for supraphysiologic doses.
Feverfew	N/A	Contraindicated; may cause uterine contractions and spontaneous abortion.	N/A	No evidence; recommend avoidance.
Magnesium	A; D (IV for >5 d)	Prolonged IV magnesium sulfate treatment associated with fetal skeletal abnormalities; oral magnesium not associated with increased risk of congenital malformations, but skeletal defects not specifically assessed.	L1 (compatible)	Safe; levels in breastmilk not affected by dietary intake.

All information in this table obtained from Micromedex, Natural Medicine, and Reprotox databases and *Hale's Medications & Mother's Milk*.

headaches during the latter two-thirds of pregnancy, it may be possible to withdraw prevention and emphasize symptomatic treatment during the first trimester.[33] Some patients make a choice to continue treatments with lower risk profiles if the baseline headache burden was high and a patient believes that managing without prevention would be intolerable. Whenever possible, medications with a higher risk burden should be converted to lower-risk medications if prevention is continued. The continuation of prevention through pregnancy is an individualized decision that should be made by the patient and physician after a thorough discussion of known safety risks. There is no evidence to suggest that treatments other than onabotulinum toxin A should be withdrawn prior to just before attempting pregnancy.

Herbs and Supplements During Pregnancy

Safety information regarding most herbal treatments, supraphysiologic doses of vitamins, and other supplements during pregnancy is lacking. Supplements are particularly challenging from a safety standpoint due to the risk of undisclosed or poorly highlighted ingredients that may be unsafe during pregnancy.[42]

Magnesium has historically been recommended as a preventive treatment during pregnancy and also has been used as an acute or rescue treatment.[43] Oral magnesium was previously in pregnancy category A. In 2014, the FDA reclassified IV magnesium sulfate used for more than 5 consecutive days as pregnancy category D after evidence of fetal skeletal malformations was discovered.[44] In the press release describing the reclassification, the FDA did not specifically address whether oral magnesium should also can be considered as having higher risk. This ruling has subsequently led to confusion about whether oral magnesium should be considered an FDA safety category A or D.[45] Databases of drugs may report either rating and attempts to contact the FDA to clarify this question were not fruitful (Rebecca Burch, MD, personal correspondence, 2018). Observational studies have not shown fetal bone abnormalities after gestational exposure to oral magnesium, but these studies were all performed before the risk associated with IV magnesium sulfate was identified. It is therefore unclear whether there is no increased risk or whether it was not effectively assessed in prior studies.

Oral magnesium has low bioavailability, and fetal serum magnesium concentrations equal maternal levels.[46,47] It, therefore, seems unlikely that oral magnesium could achieve high enough serum concentrations to compete with calcium in developing bone, as is the case for IV magnesium. An individualized approach, rather than a blanket prohibition, therefore, may be appropriate. If oral magnesium is used during pregnancy, the daily dose should be no higher than 350 mg.

MANAGEMENT OF MIGRAINE DURING LACTATION

Information about medication safety during breastfeeding is more widely available than information about use during pregnancy. Two thorough resources are the book, *Hale's Medications and Mother's Milk*, by Thomas Hale, PhD, and the online National Library of Medicine Drugs and Lactation Database.[48,49] Treatment of migraine is less restricted during lactation than during pregnancy.[50] NSAIDs, which are contraindicated during pregnancy, are first-line treatments for migraine during lactation. Triptans are also generally considered compatible with breastfeeding. Women using triptans may wish to pump and discard milk once after taking their triptan, particularly if an infant is young or low in weight. It is not clear that this is necessary, however. Of the triptans, eletriptan is the highest protein bound and, therefore, the least likely to be excreted into breastmilk.[50] Clinicians should be aware that some antiemetics, including metoclopramide, may increase milk production, whereas diphenhydramine may decrease it.

There is little overlap in the preventive medications that are contraindicated during pregnancy compared with those that are contraindicated during lactation. In general, most preventive treatments are considered low risk to moderate risk during lactation. Medications that cause sedation, such as β-blockers and tricyclic antidepressants, may be contraindicated if an infant is sleepy, had low birth weight, or has insufficient weight gain. There is no evidence for safety of onabotulinum toxin A during lactation and at this time it is recommended to avoid using this. Safety information regarding supplements during lactation is also sparse and women may not be aware of the content of such products.[51,52] The available safety information regarding treatment of migraine during lactation is summarized in **Tables 2** and **3**.

SUMMARY

Migraine is the most common cause of headache during pregnancy. Pregnancy increases the risk for dangerous causes of headache, including headaches caused by pathologic vascular processes. Any headache that is associated with neurologic signs or symptoms or is progressive and refractory to treatment, acute in onset and severe, or different from a patient's typical headaches should be evaluated. Work-up should almost always include cerebral and vascular imaging, and serum testing should be used as appropriate. Acetaminophen is the first-line symptomatic treatment during pregnancy, and there is growing evidence supporting the use of triptans rather than butalbital combination analgesics as second-line treatment. Propranolol is the preferred preventive treatment, and amitriptyline and verapamil also may be considered. Treatment of migraine during lactation is typically less restrictive than during pregnancy.

REFERENCES

1. Burch R, Rizzoli P, Loder E. The prevalence and impact of migraine and severe headache in the United States: figures and trends from government health studies. Headache 2018;58(4):496–505.
2. Buse DC, Loder EW, Gorman JA, et al. Sex differences in the prevalence, symptoms, and associated features of migraine, probable migraine and other severe headache: results of the American Migraine Prevalence and Prevention (AMPP) Study. Headache 2013;53(8):1278–99.
3. IHS Classification. ICHD-3 The international classification of headache disorders 3rd edition. ICHD-3 The international classification of headache disorders 3rd edition. Available at: https://www.ichd-3.org/. Accessed June 2, 2018.
4. Robbins MS, Farmakidis C, Dayal AK, et al. Acute headache diagnosis in pregnant women: a hospital-based study. Neurology 2015;85(12):1024–30.
5. Raffaelli B, Siebert E, Körner J, et al. Characteristics and diagnoses of acute headache in pregnant women - a retrospective cross-sectional study. J Headache Pain 2017;18(1):114.
6. Negro A, Delaruelle Z, Ivanova TA, et al. Headache and pregnancy: a systematic review. J Headache Pain 2017;18(1):106.
7. Bushnell CD, Jamison M, James AH. Migraines during pregnancy linked to stroke and vascular diseases: US population based case-control study. BMJ 2009;338: b664.
8. Goldszmidt E, Kern R, Chaput A, et al. The incidence and etiology of postpartum headaches: a prospective cohort study. Can J Anaesth 2005;52(9):971–7.

9. Vgontzas A, Robbins MS. A hospital based retrospective study of acute post-partum headache. Headache 2018. https://doi.org/10.1111/head.13279.

10. Klein JP, Hsu L. Neuroimaging during pregnancy. Semin Neurol 2011;31(4): 361–73.

11. Frederick IO, Qiu C, Enquobahrie DA, et al. Lifetime prevalence and correlates of migraine among women in a pacific northwest pregnancy cohort study. Headache 2014;54(4):675–85.

12. Wright GD, Patel MK. Focal migraine and pregnancy. Br Med J 1986;293(6561): 1557–8.

13. Lebedeva ER, Gurary NM, Gilev DV, et al. Prospective testing of ICHD-3 beta diagnostic criteria for migraine with aura and migraine with typical aura in patients with transient ischemic attacks. Cephalalgia 2018;38(3):561–7.

14. Sances G, Granella F, Nappi RE, et al. Course of migraine during pregnancy and postpartum: a prospective study. Cephalalgia 2003;23(3):197–205.

15. Granella F, Sances G, Zanferrari C, et al. Migraine without aura and reproductive life events: a clinical epidemiological study in 1300 women. Headache 1993; 33(7):385–9.

16. Hypertension in pregnancy - ACOG. Available at: https://www.acog.org/Clinical-Guidance-and-Publications/Task_Force_and_Work_Group-Reports/Hypertension-in-Pregnancy. Accessed June 2, 2018.

17. Douglas KA, Redman CW. Eclampsia in the United Kingdom. BMJ 1994; 309(6966):1395–400.

18. Ducros A, Wolff V. The typical thunderclap headache of reversible cerebral vaso-constriction syndrome and its various triggers. Headache 2016;56(4):657–73.

19. Ducros A. Reversible cerebral vasoconstriction syndrome. Lancet Neurol 2012; 11(10):906–17.

20. Cantu-Brito C, Arauz A, Aburto Y, et al. Cerebrovascular complications during pregnancy and postpartum: clinical and prognosis observations in 240 Hispanic women. Eur J Neurol 2011;18(6):819–25.

21. Edlow JA, Caplan LR, O'Brien K, et al. Diagnosis of acute neurological emergencies in pregnant and post-partum women. Lancet Neurol 2013;12(2):175–85.

22. Coutinho JM, Stam J, Canhão P, et al. Cerebral venous thrombosis in the absence of headache. Stroke 2015;46(1):245–7.

23. Coutinho JM, Ferro JM, Canhão P, et al. Cerebral venous and sinus thrombosis in women. Stroke 2009;40(7):2356–61.

24. Digre KB, Varner MW, Corbett JJ. Pseudotumor cerebri and pregnancy. Neurology 1984;34(6):721–9.

25. Mathew M, Salahuddin A, Mathew NR, et al. Idiopathic intracranial hypertension presenting as postpartum headache. Neurosciences (Riyadh) 2016;21(1):52–5.

26. Friedman DI. Idiopathic intracranial hypertension. Curr Pain Headache Rep 2007; 11(1):62–8.

27. Kesler A, Kupferminc M. Idiopathic intracranial hypertension and pregnancy. Clin Obstet Gynecol 2013;56(2):389–96.

28. Choi PT, Galinski SE, Takeuchi L, et al. PDPH is a common complication of neuraxial blockade in parturients: a meta-analysis of obstetrical studies. Can J Anaesth 2003;50(5):460–9.

29. Banks S, Paech M, Gurrin L. An audit of epidural blood patch after accidental dural puncture with a Tuohy needle in obstetric patients. Int J Obstet Anesth 2001; 10(3):172–6.

30. Rist PM, Diener H-C, Kurth T, et al. Migraine, migraine aura, and cervical artery dissection: a systematic review and meta-analysis. Cephalalgia 2011;31(8): 886–96.

31. Millstine D, Chen CY, Bauer B. Complementary and integrative medicine in the management of headache. BMJ 2017;357:j1805.

32. Evaluation CFD, Research. labeling - pregnancy and lactation labeling (drugs) final rule. Available at: https://www.fda.gov/Drugs/DevelopmentApprovalProcess/ DevelopmentResources/Labeling/ucm093307.htm. Accessed June 2, 2018.

33. Silberstein SD. Headaches in pregnancy. J Headache Pain 2005;6(4):172–4.

34. Baigi K, Stewart WF. Headache and migraine: a leading cause of absenteeism. Handb Clin Neurol 2015;131:447–63.

35. Babu GR, Murthy GVS, Singh N, et al. Sociodemographic and medical risk factors associated with antepartum depression. Front Public Health 2018;6:127.

36. Bruehl S, Chung OY, Jirjis JN, et al. Prevalence of clinical hypertension in patients with chronic pain compared to nonpain general medical patients. Clin J Pain 2005;21(2):147–53.

37. Nakhai-Pour HR, Broy P, Sheehy O, et al. Use of nonaspirin nonsteroidal anti-inflammatory drugs during pregnancy and the risk of spontaneous abortion. CMAJ 2011;183(15):1713–20.

38. Marchenko A, Etwel F, Olutunfese O, et al. Pregnancy outcome following prenatal exposure to triptan medications: a meta-analysis. Headache 2015;55(4): 490–501.

39. Marmura MJ, Silberstein SD, Schwedt TJ. The acute treatment of migraine in adults: the american headache society evidence assessment of migraine pharmacotherapies. Headache 2015;55(1):3–20.

40. Childress KMS, Dothager C, Gavard JA, et al. Metoclopramide and diphenhydramine: a randomized controlled trial of a treatment for headache in pregnancy when acetaminophen alone is ineffective (MAD Headache Study). Am J Perinatol 2018. https://doi.org/10.1055/s-0038-1646952.

41. Brin MF, Kirby RS, Slavotinek A, et al. Pregnancy outcomes following exposure to onabotulinumtoxinA. Pharmacoepidemiol Drug Saf 2015;25(2):179–87.

42. Gabay M, Smith JA, Chavez ML, et al. White paper on natural products. Pharmacotherapy 2017;37(1):e1–15.

43. Airola G, Allais G, Gabellari IC, et al. Non-pharmacological management of migraine during pregnancy. Neurol Sci 2010;31(S1):63–5.

44. [No title]. Available at: https://www.fda.gov/downloads/Drugs/DrugSafety/ UCM353335.pdf. Accessed June 2, 2018.

45. Wells RE, Turner DP, Lee M, et al. Managing migraine during pregnancy and lactation. Curr Neurol Neurosci Rep 2016;16(4):40.

46. Uysal N, Kizildag S, Yuce Z, et al. Timeline (Bioavailability) of magnesium compounds in hours: which magnesium compound works best? Biol Trace Elem Res 2018. https://doi.org/10.1007/s12011-018-1351-9.

47. Osada H, Watanabe Y, Nishimura Y, et al. Profile of trace element concentrations in the feto-placental unit in relation to fetal growth. Acta Obstet Gynecol Scand 2002;81(10):931–7.

48. Drugs and Lactation Database (LactMed). Available at: https://toxnet.nlm.nih. gov/newtoxnet/lactmed.htm. Accessed June 3, 2018.

49. Hale TW. Hale's medications & mothers' milk: 2019. New York: Springer Publishing Company; 2018.

50. Hutchinson S, Marmura MJ, Calhoun A, et al. Use of common migraine treatments in breast-feeding women: a summary of recommendations. Headache 2013;53(4):614–27.
51. Amer MR, Cipriano GC, Venci JV, et al. Safety of popular herbal supplements in lactating women. J Hum Lact 2015;31(3):348–53.
52. Bettiol A, Lombardi N, Marconi E, et al. The use of complementary and alternative medicines during breastfeeding: results from the Herbal supplements in Breast-feeding InvesTigation (HaBIT). Br J Clin Pharmacol 2018. https://doi.org/10.1111/bcp.13639.
53. Micromedex. Available at: https://www.micromedexsolutions.com/. Accessed October 17, 2018.
54. Natural Medicines Comprehensive Database. Available at: https://naturalmedicines.therapeuticresearch.com/. Accessed October 17, 2018.
55. Reprotox. Available at: https://reprotox.org/. Accessed October 17, 2018.

Epilepsy in Pregnancy

Cynthia Harden, MD[a],*, Christine Lu, MD[b]

KEYWORDS

- Epilepsy • Pregnancy • Contraception • Infertility • Teratogenicity
- Labor and delivery • Breastfeeding

KEY POINTS

- Discussions about contraception and pregnancy with women with epilepsy should occur at every visit.
- Women with epilepsy should contact their provider if they become pregnant and should not stop antiepileptic drugs on their own.
- Clinicians should advise all women of childbearing potential to take at least 0.4 mg of folic acid daily to optimize cognitive outcomes in offspring.
- Valproate should be avoided for women of childbearing potential due to the high risk of teratogenesis. Lamotrigine and levetiracetam are the safest antiseizure medications for pregnancy.
- Breastfeeding should be encouraged for women with epilepsy.

INTRODUCTION

Epilepsy is a prevalent, chronic, and serious neurologic disease for which treatment usually must be maintained during pregnancy. Therefore, the teratogenic risk of antiepileptic drugs (AEDs) is an obvious concern but it is one among many. Most management strategies surrounding pregnancy involve counseling, therefore this article is organized to address the common questions posed by women with epilepsy (WWE) in a naturalistic and chronologic sequence, as would be encountered in an office visit.

CONTRACEPTION

The choice of contraception for WWE is complex due to interactions between enzyme-inducing AEDs (EIAEDs) and hormonal contraceptives. Because about 65%

Disclosure Statement: The authors report no disclosures.

[a] The Head of the Therapeutic Area of Epilepsy for Xenon Pharmaceuticals, Inc, 332 East 14th Street, New York, NY 10003, USA; [b] Department of Neurology, Mount Sinai Downtown, 10 Union Square East Suite 5D, New York, NY 10003, USA
* Corresponding author.
E-mail address: clouish17@gmail.com

of pregnancies are unplanned, discussion regarding contraception, until when or if pregnancy is sought, should occur at every office visit.[1] Ideally, WWE should be counseled regarding the choice of contraceptive and its interaction with AEDs before they become sexually active. Two major concerns are hormonal contraceptive failure and reduced AED efficacy, both of which are due to pharmacokinetic interactions between these 2 medication types through cytochrome (CYP)P450-P3A4 (CYP3A4).[2]

AEDs with CYP3A4 enzyme-inducing properties, including carbamazepine, oxcarbazepine, felbamate, phenytoin, primidone, topiramate, perampanel, and phenobarbital decrease circulating levels of estrogen and the progestins (synthetic forms of progesterone) in oral contraceptives because these hormones are substrates for CYP3A4.[3] Although clear evidence for oral contraceptive failure with EIAEDs has been scant, a principle-proving study has been performed. In a double-blind, randomized, crossover trial, ovulation rates were much higher during carbamazepine administration compared with placebo in women taking a combined oral contraceptive (COC).[4] These findings can be extrapolated to a potential for contraceptive failure with all EIAEDs. This risk cannot be mitigated by a COC containing a higher dose of estrogen because only the progestin component of the COC provides contraception, primarily via inhibition of ovulation. The low-dose progestin-only formulations may not consistently inhibit ovulation due to the low dose they deliver but may prevent pregnancy through peripheral mechanisms, the most important of which is by thickening cervical mucus and preventing sperm passage.

WWE taking EIAEDS should be advised to use condoms with spermicide, depot medroxyprogesterone injections, or intrauterine devices (**Table 1**). AEDs that have no interactions with hormonal contraceptives and pose no risk of contraceptive failure are valproic acid, vigabatrin, gabapentin, tiagabine, levetiracetam, zonisamide, ethosuximide, and benzodiazepines, including clobazam and clonazepam.[5]

In the other direction of pharmacologic interaction, the estrogenic component of COCs can lower lamotrigine levels by 40% to 60%, increasing the risk of breakthrough seizures. Estradiol induces uridine-diphosphate glucuronosyl transferase (UGT), which catalyzes glucuronidation, the major metabolic pathway for lamotrigine.[6] Therefore, lamotrigine levels should be carefully monitored before and after starting a COC, and doses adjusted accordingly, potentially by up to 50%. Lamotrigine levels are not

Table 1
Choice of contraception

Form of Contraception	Risk of Contraceptive Failure
COC pill (estrogen and progesterone)	Contraceptive efficacy lower with hepatic enzyme-inducing drugs: carbamazepine, oxcarbazepine, felbamate, phenytoin, primidone, topiramate, perampanel, and phenobarbital
Progesterone-only pill	Contraceptive efficacy lower with hepatic enzyme-inducing drugs and likely with lamotrigine
Depot injection	Not affected
Implant	Similar effects to COC
Dermal patch	Similar effects to COC
Vaginal ring	Similar effects to COC
Intrauterine device	Not affected
Mechanical barrier (diaphragm, cup, male or female condom)	Not affected

affected by the progestins of COCs. However, lamotrigine induces the clearance of progestins with a resultant decrease in progestin level of approximately 20%. Therefore, although the progestin-only OC may seem to be reasonable for women taking lamotrigine, the risk of contraceptive failure would predictably be increased with this combination as well.

UGT glucuronidation is also important for valproate and eslicarbazepine metabolism, and COCs clearly reduce valproate levels by 20% to 40%. There is a potential for COCs to also lower eslicarbazepine levels. These latter 2 AED interactions with COCs have not generally been clinically important.

INFERTILITY

Birth rates among WWE are lower than the general population. A Finland registry comprising 12,058 subjects over 39 years, 222 of whom were identified to have epilepsy, found fewer children among adults with active epilepsy.[7] However, low birth rates do not translate directly into infertility. Psychosocial contributors, such as low marriage rates and less desire to have children, are reported in WWE.[8] The direct relationship between epilepsy and infertility remain unclear.

A recent prospective observational trial enrolled WWE who are actively seeking pregnancy. Sexual activity and menstrual cycle were matched to controls, thus eliminating some of the psychosocial factors of low birth rate. In this study, no difference was found between the epilepsy and control group in pregnancy rates (60.7% vs 60.2%, respectively), or median time to pregnancy (6 months vs 9 months, respectively) at 1 year.[9] However, nearly all subjects in this study were taking either lamotrigine or levetiracetam monotherapy, which is important to note when considering the generalizability of this study. Only a few subjects were taking EIAEDs that are known to alter endogenous (as well as exogenous) reproductive hormone levels. Therefore, with the use of EIAEDS, an effect on fertility could be postulated.

Indeed, in a naturalistic observational study, the use of phenobarbital and polytherapy in WWE trying to conceive were risk factors for infertility. In this study, the number of AEDs taken was positively associated with a higher rate of infertility (1 AED 31.8%, 2 AEDs 40.7%, and 3 or more AEDs 60.3%). Use of 3 or more AEDs has an odds ratio as high as 17.9. Half of the women who took phenobarbital were unable to conceive over several years of attempt at conception. Furthermore, the overall association of EIAEDs with infertility risk is supported by the findings.[10]

RISK OF ADVERSE OUTCOMES IN THE MOTHER

Pregnancy does not generally alter the frequency of seizures in WWE. Although percentages vary across studies, in approximately 60% of patients, seizure frequency is similar to that of the prepregnancy baseline, whereas 15% experience an increase in frequency and 15% experience a decrease.[11] If the patient was seizure-free for 1 year before pregnancy, it is very likely (80%) that she will continue to remain seizure-free during pregnancy.[12] Rates of status epilepticus in pregnant WWE are comparable to the annual frequency of 1.6% in the general epilepsy population.[13]

Other maternal pregnancy-related complications, such as gestational hypertension and preeclampsia, may be increased in WWE with an odds ratio of about 1.5, based on a Norwegian population-based registry.[14] AED use contributed to the overall risk.[15] However, no difference in incidence of these complications between WWE and controls was found in a prospective controlled study of 179 pregnancies in WWE.[16]

Therefore, the risk of these complications may be slightly increased but is certainly close to the range of the expected incidence.

Maternal mortality is 10-fold higher in WWE than the general population, most of which is presumably due to sudden unexpected death in epilepsy (SUDEP), which is commonly known by its acronym.[17] In 1 report, half of the epilepsy-related deaths (79% from SUDEP) occurred in patients who were on lamotrigine as monotherapy, highlighting the importance of monitoring drug levels that are affected by hormonal changes (see later discussion).[18]

RISK OF ADVERSE OUTCOMES IN THE FETUS

About 24,000 babies are born to WWE in the United States each year. There is an increased risk of small for gestational age birth weight and head circumference in association with AED use.[19,20] Seizures during pregnancy have not been linked to immediate fetal complications, except in cases of maternal hypoxia, in which fetal bradycardia has been documented, which is reversible with the termination of seizure activity.[21] However, some studies reported an increased risk of preterm birth in women with untreated epilepsy compared with women without epilepsy.[22] This trend is observed in a separate study in a subgroup of WWE who smoke.[23] Therefore, it is especially important to counsel WWE regarding smoking during pregnancy.

The most well-known and documented AED teratogenicity is valproate causing neural tube defects. The risk of valproate causing major congenital malformations (MCMs) is 10% and is clearly dose-associated. Daily doses of 1500 mg per day or greater are associated with a risk of 24%, whereas doses of 700 mg per day or less carry a risk of 5% to 6%.[24] These malformations are serious and consist of midline defects such as spina bifida, hypospadias, and brain malformations in utero, the latter of which may not be compatible with a viable pregnancy. Limb defects such as radial ray malformations also occur. The risk of neural tube defects, cardiac malformations, and facial clefts in general occur at a higher rate with in utero AED exposure and are considered a drug class effect; however, the risk with valproate is significantly higher than with other AEDs. Further, valproate exposure in utero is associated with an increased risk of autism or autism spectrum disorder, even when maternal epilepsy is not present.[25] Consistent with this association, valproate exposure in utero was found to cause reduced cognitive outcomes in children tested at 6 years of age; this risk was also related to dose. In general, the comparator arms of phenytoin, carbamazepine, and lamotrigine in this study were associated with expected cognitive outcomes in exposed offspring. Importantly, in this study, folic acid use of at least 0.4 mg per day and breast-feeding (see later discussion) were both associated with improved cognitive outcomes. The adverse effect of valproate was nearly normalized to the expected range of cognitive scores in the valproate-exposed but breastfed group.[26]

Other important and specific MCMs are cardiac defects with phenobarbital, the first AED found to be teratogenic from the North American AED Pregnancy Registry, with an overall risk of MCMs of 6%, and cardiac defects with topiramate, which carries a risk of 4%, with facial clefts as the specific adverse outcome.[27] With topiramate and zonisamide exposure, there is also a clear risk of low birth weight.[28] Lamotrigine, carbamazepine, phenytoin, and levetiracetam, the other AEDs evaluated in this study, were associated with a teratogenic risk for MCMs between 2% and 3%, rates of which do not clearly differentiate from the risk in the general population.[27] From a recent Cochrane review of this topic, levetiracetam and lamotrigine were found to carry the lowest teratogenic risk.[29] These considerations must be balanced with the risk of seizures also present with their use if the levels decrease to a nonprotective range.

The US Food and Drug Administration (FDA) category of pregnancy risk for AEDs is presented in **Table 2**. While these categories still stand for the AEDs listed, as of June 30th, 2015 the FDA is no longer using these letter categories to denote pregnancy risk. Pregnancy risk for newly approved medications will include a brief discussion of registry information when available, lactation information and available clinical information regarding contraception and infertility. Drugs previously approved will be gradually changed over to the updated presentation of risk.

The risk of the child developing epilepsy in life depends mainly on the type of epilepsy in the mother. Patients with hereditary epilepsy syndromes should be counseled accordingly. An increased incidence of epilepsy is associated with decreasing gestational age and birth weight. Children born at 22 to 32 weeks with a birth weight of less than 2000 g have a 5-fold increase in risk of developing epilepsy in the first year of life compared with children born 39 to 41 weeks with birth weight of 3000 to 3999 g.[30]

PRACTICAL MANAGEMENT OF ANTIEPILEPTIC DRUGS

WWE should discuss plans of pregnancy with their health care provider, and providers should be open to each individual's choice regarding risks and benefits of AEDs. However, clinicians should communicate 1 clear message to their patients: if they discover they are pregnant, do not stop taking AEDs and call their provider to discuss next steps in management. Pregnant WWE are twice as likely to stop AED as nonpregnant WWE[31] and it is a fundamental principle of care that uncontrolled epilepsy poses a major health risk to the mother as well as the fetus.

Before conception, seizure control should be optimized because seizure frequency in the previous year is comparable to that of pregnancy.[31] However, this predictor depends on the AED level not decreasing more than 35% of the preconception level, which may be challenging due to changes in pregnancy such as increased drug clearance, volume expansion, and hormone fluctuations.[32] The American Academy of Neurology (AAN) recommends monitoring AED levels during pregnancy.[33] Therefore, it is important to first establish a therapeutic range in the preconception stage to

Table 2	
US Food and Drug Administration pregnancy categories of antiepileptic drugs	
FDA Category C drugs	FDA Category D drugs
• Acetazolamide	• Carbamazepine
• Clobazam	• Clonazepam
• Ethosuximide	• Phenobarbital
• Felbamate	• Phenytoin
• Gabapentin	• Topiramate
• Lamotrigine	• Valproate
• Levetiracetam	
• Oxcarbazepine	
• Tiagabine	
• Vigabatrin	
• Zonisamide	

FDA category C: Animal reproduction studies have shown an adverse effect on the fetus and there are no adequate and well-controlled studies in humans but potential benefits may warrant use of the drug in pregnant women despite potential risks. FDA category D: There is positive evidence of human fetal risk based on adverse reaction data from investigational or marketing experience or studies in humans but potential benefits may warrant use of the drug in pregnant women despite potential risks. There are currently no FDA Category A or B AEDs.

eliminate interindividual variations. Levels may be checked in each trimester and in the postpartum period.[34] Lamotrigine and oxcarbazepine levels should be followed more closely, at monthly intervals or even more frequently, owing to their marked increase in clearance in the setting of high estrogen levels. Levetiracetam and zonisamide also decrease markedly during pregnancy owing to increased renal clearance, and should be followed closely.

In patients with controlled epilepsy, attempts should be made to reduce the AED dose to the lowest therapeutic range during preconception. Polytherapy should also be avoided because it likely increases the risk of MCMs.[35] In the UK Epilepsy and Pregnancy Registry of 3607 cases, the risk of malformations with polytherapy is 6.0%, as opposed to 3.7% with monotherapy.[36] The risk is especially higher with the use of valproate.[37]

The AAN and Epilepsy Foundation encourage all WWE to take folic acid supplementation, possibly at a higher dose (4 mg) than what is recommended for the general population (0.4 mg).[33,38] Folic acid is a B vitamin involved in the synthesis of purines, which are required for DNA formation, and low levels are associated with reduced growth and anemia. Infants of women on folic acid antagonists (dihydrofolate reductase inhibitors), such as phenytoin, phenobarbital, or carbamazepine, during the first trimester are at higher risk of MCMs with a relative risk of 3.4.[39] Folic acid deficiency has also been implicated in neural tube defects in the general population, which is a known adverse outcome with the use of valproate and carbamazepine during pregnancy.[40] Finally, WWE on hepatic EIAEDs are at increased risk of low folic acid by up to 90%.[41] Therefore, although there are no randomized controlled trials studying the effects of folic acid in preventing MCMs in WWE, the protective effect of folic acid supplementation on cognitive outcome has been shown.[26] Therefore, all WWE should be encouraged to take at least 0.4 mg of folic acid daily.

LABOR AND DELIVERY

Seizures during delivery occur in about 2% of WWE,[42] with greater risk to those who have subtherapeutic AED levels.[43] Maternal seizures in labor may result in prolonged uterine contractions with slowing of fetal heart rate.[44] A Swedish study of 1,429,652 births, 5373 of which were births to 3586 WWE, showed that WWE are at risk of adverse delivery outcomes, including peripartum infection, placental abruption, induction, and elective cesarean section, after adjusting for psychosocial confounders.[45] Similarly, in a US study of 20,449,532 delivery hospitalizations, 69,385 of which were of WWE, there is a higher risk of preeclampsia, preterm labor, increased cesarean delivery, and prolonged hospital stay (>6 days), as well as a 10-fold increased risk of mortality (adjusted odds ratio 11.46).[46] Thus, although epilepsy is not an indication for cesarean delivery, home births are highly discouraged. WWE are recommended to deliver in a hospital setting and take their AEDs regularly through labor.

BREASTFEEDING

Breastfeeding provides many benefits for the infant, including nutrition and immunoprotection, as well as social development. Most concerns with breastfeeding lie in the potential transfer of AEDs through breast milk and their side effects. However, few studies have established minimal, if any, disadvantage to breastfeeding in women with treated epilepsy. Continuous breastfeeding in the first 6 months of life is associated with improved outcome in fine motor, gross motor, and social skills in a Norwegian Mother and Child Cohort Study (n = 78,744).[47] In another study of 181 children with mothers on AED monotherapy, in which approximately half of the children were

Table 3
Counseling

Stage	
All women diagnosed with epilepsy • I have a boyfriend and I am sexually active; what do I need to know or do? • What kind of birth control should I use? • I am planning to have children in the future. What should I do?	• Ask if the patient is sexually active. Supplement folic acid. • Depending on the AED, the patient's contraception options should be discussed. • Encourage the patient to discuss family planning with the provider in advance and to run all medication changes by the provider.
Preconception • Will I have trouble getting pregnant? • How do I adjust my medicine before pregnancy? Can I come off my medicines? • What vitamins do I need to take? • What tests do I need to take?	• Reassure the patient that fertility is the same as the general population in WWE actively seeking to become pregnant. • Optimize seizure control and AED regimen. Use as few AEDs at as low doses as possible. Patients with uncontrolled epilepsy should not discontinue their AEDs. • Supplement folic acid if not already taking. • Establish therapeutic AED levels.
Pregnancy • Will my seizures increase? • What should I do if I have a seizure? • Does having a seizure affect my baby? • How is my seizure medicine going to affect my baby? • Do I need to have a cesarean section? • Can I have a home birth?	• Reassure patient that seizure frequency is usually similar to preconception. • General seizure management remains the same. AED levels should be checked at least each trimester. If a patient has a breakthrough seizure, try to identify triggers, such as decreased absorption of AEDs due to hyperemesis gravidarum. Discuss dose increase or addition of AEDs with patient based on risks and benefits. • There is little evidence to suggest that seizures per se in the mother adversely affect the fetus except in prolonged seizures or with direct trauma. • MCMs are rare but more common than the general population. Risks and benefits of AED treatment should be discussed with the patient and the decision made based on her preference. • Epilepsy is not an indication for a cesarean section but the obstetrician should be aware of the diagnosis and be prepared. • Home birth should be discouraged due to potential seizures during labor.
Postpartum and breastfeeding • Can I breastfeed? • Can I hold the baby? • Will I need help to take care of my newborn baby?	• Encourage patient to breastfeed. • In patients with uncontrolled epilepsy, a safety strap is recommended while holding the baby. • WWE should obtain as much help as frequently as they can to promote adequate self-care, including sleep, stress reduction, and mood.

breastfed for a mean of 7.2 months, breastfed children exhibited higher IQ at 6 years of age, with no observed side effects.[48] Breastfeeding also reduces the risk of the child developing epilepsy at 1 year of age in a dose-dependent fashion; children who were breastfed longer had decreasing risk.[49] WWE should be reassured and encouraged to breastfeed.

In considering AEDs, lipophilic drugs have a high penetrance into breast milk, whereas protein-bound drugs have lower penetrance. Phenytoin, valproate, and carbamazepine are moderately to highly protein-bound and have a low milk to plasma ratio.[50] Very few case reports of adverse reaction are documented.[51] Most other AEDs have either a low penetrance into breast milk, low infant serum drug levels, or rare side effects. Two exceptions are phenobarbital and benzodiazepines. Due to their long half-lives (diazepam has a half-life of 30 hours in newborns), drugs can accumulate, causing drowsiness and poor weight gain. Careful monitoring is warranted.[50]

Counseling strategies based on common questions posed by patients and families are presented in **Table 3**.

REFERENCES

1. Herzog AG, Mandel HB, Cahill KE, et al. Predictors of unintended pregnancy in women with epilepsy. Neurology 2017;88:728–33.
2. Zupanc ML. Antiepileptic drugs and hormonal contraceptives in adolescent women with epilepsy. Neurology 2006;66:S37–45.
3. Brodie MJ, Mintzer S, Pack AM, et al. Enzyme induction with antiepileptic drugs: cause for concern? Epilepsia 2013;54:11–27.
4. Davis AR, Westhoff CL, Stanczyk FZ. Carbamazepine co-administration with an oral contraceptive: effects on steroid pharmacokinetics, ovulation, and bleeding. Epilepsia 2011;52:243–7.
5. O'Brien MD, Guillebaud J. Contraception for women with epilepsy. Epilepsia 2006;47:1419–22.
6. Reddy DS. Clinical pharmacokinetic interactions between antiepileptic drugs and hormonal contraceptives. Expert Rev Clin Pharmacol 2011;3:183–92.
7. Lofgren E, Pouta A, von Wendt L, et al. Epilepsy in the northern Finland birth cohort 1966 with special reference to fertility. Epilepsy Behav 2009;14:102–7.
8. Crawford P, Hudson S. Understanding the information needs of women with epilepsy at different lifestages: results of the 'Ideal world' survey. Seizure 2003;12:502–7.
9. Pennel PB, French JA, Harden CL, et al. Fertility and birth outcomes in women with epilepsy seeking pregnancy. JAMA Neurol 2018;75(8):962–9.
10. Sukumaran SC, Sarma PS, Thomas SV. Polytherapy increases the risk of infertility in women with epilepsy. Neurology 2010;75(15):1351–5.
11. The EURAP Study Group. Seizure control and treatment in pregnancy. Neurology 2006;66:354–60.
12. Vajda FJ, Hitchcock A, Graham J, et al. Seizure control in antiepileptic drug-treated pregnancy. Epilepsia 2008;49:172–6.
13. Harden CL, Hopp J, Ting TY, et al. Practice parameter update: management issues for women with epilepsy—focus on pregnancy (an evidence-based review): obstetrical complications and change in seizure frequency. Neurology 2009;73:126–32.
14. Borthern I, Eide M, Veiby G, et al. Complications during pregnancy in women with epilepsy: population-based cohort study. BJOG 2009;116:1736–42.

15. Borthern I, Gilhus NE. Pregnancy complications in patients with epilepsy. Curr Opin Obstet Gynecol 2012;24:78–83.
16. Viinikainen K, Heinonen S, Eriksson K, et al. Community-based, prospective, controlled study of obstetric and neonatal outcome of 179 pregnancies in women with epilepsy. Epilepsia 2006;47:186–92.
17. Adab N, Ayres J, Baker G, et al. The longer term outcomes of children born to mothers with epilepsy. J Neurol Neurosurg Psychiatry 2004;75:1575–83.
18. Edey S, Moran N, Nashef L. SUDEP and epilepsy-related mortality in pregnancy. Epilepsia 2014;55:e72–4.
19. Borgelt LM, Hart FM, Bainbridge JL. Epilepsy during pregnancy: focus on management strategies. Int J Womens Health 2016;8:505–17.
20. Hernandez-Diaz S, McElrath TF, Pennell PB, et al. Fetal growth and premature delivery in pregnant women on antiepileptic drugs. Ann Neurol 2017;82:457–65.
21. Sibai BM. Diagnosis, prevention, and management of eclampsia. Obstet Gynecol 2005;105:402–10.
22. Kilic D, Pedersen H, Kjaersgaard MIS, et al. Birth outcomes after prenatal exposure to antiepileptic drugs—a population-based study. Epilepsia 2014;55:1714–21.
23. Hvas CL, Henriksen TB, østergaard JR, et al. Epilepsy and pregnancy: effect of antiepileptic drugs and lifestyle on birthweight. BJOG 2000;107:896–902.
24. Tomson T, Battino D, Bonizzoni E, et al. Dose-dependent teratogenicity of valproate in mono- and polytherapy: an observational study. Neurology 2015;85:866–72.
25. Christensen J, Gronborg TK, Sorensen MJ, et al. Prenatal valproate exposure and risk of autism spectrum disorders and childhood autism. JAMA 2013;309:1696–703.
26. Meador KJ, Baker GA, Browning N, et al. Fetal antiepileptic drug exposure and cognitive outcomes at age 6 years (NEAD study): a prospective observational study. Lancet Neurol 2013;12:244–52.
27. Hernandez-Diaz S, Smith CR, Shen A, et al. Comparative safety of antiepileptic drugs during pregnancy. Neurology 2012;78:1692–9.
28. Hernandez-Diaz S, Mittendorf R, Smith CR, et al. Association between topiramate and zonisamide use during pregnancy and low birth weight. Obstet Gynecol 2014;123:21–8.
29. Weston J, Bromley R, Jackson CF, et al. Monotherapy treatment of epilepsy in pregnancy: congenital malformation outcomes in the child. Cochrane Database Syst Rev 2016;(11):CD010224.
30. Sun Y, Vestergaard M, Pedersen CB, et al. Gestational age, birth weight, intrauterine gowth and risk for epilepsy. Am J Epidemiol 2008;167:262–70.
31. Man SL, Petersen I, Thompson M, et al. Antiepileptic drugs during pregnancy in primary care: a UK population based study. PLoS One 2012;7:e52339.
32. Reisinger TL, Newman M, Loring DW, et al. Antiepileptic drug clearance and seizure frequency during pregnancy in women with epilepsy. Epilepsy Behav 2013;29:13–8.
33. Harden CL, Pennell PB, Koppel BS, et al. Practice parameter update: management issues for women with epilepsy-focus on pregnancy (an evidence-based review): vitamin K, folic acid, blood levels, and breastfeeding. Neurology 2009;73:142–9.
34. Adab N. Therapeutic monitoring of antiepileptic drugs during pregnancy and in the postpartum period: is it useful? CNS Drugs 2006;20:791–800.

35. Pennell PB. Antiepilptic drugs during pregnancy: what is known and which AEDs seem to be safest? Epilepsia 2008;49(Suppl 9):43–55.

36. Morrow J, Russell A, Guthrie E, et al. Malformation risks of antiepileptic drugs in pregnancy: a prospective study from the UK epilepsy and pregnancy register. J Neurol Neurosurg Psychiatry 2006;77:193–8.

37. Artama M, Auvinen A, Raudaskoski T, et al. Antiepileptic drug use of women with epilepsy and congenital malformations in offspring. Neurology 2005;64:1874–8.

38. Epilepsy Foundation. Folic acid. 2018. Available at: https://www.epilepsy.com/living-epilepsy/women/all-women/folic-acid. Accessed May 30, 2018.

39. Hernandez-Diaz S, Werler MM, Walker AM, et al. Folic acid antagonists during pregnancy and the risk of birth defects. N Engl J Med 2000;343:1608–14.

40. Yerby MS. Management issues for women with epilepsy neural tube defects and folic acid supplementation. Neurology 2003;61:S23–6.

41. Morrell MJ. Folic acid and epilepsy. Epilepsy Curr 2002;2:31–4.

42. Sveberg L, Svalheim S, Tauboll E. The impact of seizures on pregnancy and delivery. Seizure 2015;28:35–8.

43. Katz JM, Devinsky O. Primary generalized epilepsy: a risk factor for seizures in labor and delivery? Seizure 2003;12:217–9.

44. Nei M, Daly S, Liporace J. A maternal complex partial seizure in labor can affect fetal heart rate. Neurology 1998;51:904–6.

45. Razaz N, Tomson T, Wikstrom A-K, et al. Association between pregnancy and perinatal outcomes among women with epilepsy. JAMA Neurol 2017;74:983–91.

46. MacDonald SC, Bateman BT, McElrath TF, et al. Mortality and morbidity during delivery hospitalization among pregnant women with epilepsy in the United States. JAMA Neurol 2015;72:981–8.

47. Veiby G, Engelsen BA, Gilhus NE. Early child development and exposure to antiepileptic drugs prenatally and through breastfeeding. JAMA Neurol 2013;70:1367–74.

48. Meador KJ, Baker GA, Browning N, et al. Breastfeeding in children of women taking antiepileptic drugs: cognitive outcomes at age 6 years. JAMA Pediatr 2014;168:729–36.

49. Drugs and Lactation Database (LactMed). 2018. Available at: https://toxnet.nlm.nih.gov/newtoxnet/lactmed.htm. Accessed May 30, 2018.

50. Sun Y, Vestergaard M, Christensen J, et al. Breastfeeding and risk of epilepsy in childhood: a birth cohort study. J Pediatr 2011;158:924–9.

51. Veiby G, Bjork M, Engelsen BA, et al. Epilepsy and recommendations for breastfeeding. Seizure 2015;28:57–65.

Pituitary Disorders in Pregnancy

Whitney W. Woodmansee, MD

KEYWORDS

- Pregnancy • Pituitary adenoma • Hypophysitis • Sheehan syndrome
- Hypopituitarism

KEY POINTS

- Normal pregnancy is associated with pituitary enlargement and changes in pituitary hormonal physiology.
- Abnormal pituitary function can cause infertility, with hyperprolactinemia being one of the most common causes of central hypogonadism.
- Pituitary adenomas are relatively common and all patients should be evaluated for mass effects and pituitary hormonal hypofunction and hyperfunction.
- Pituitary hormonal deficiencies must be adequately replaced before and during pregnancy.
- Women with pituitary adenomas can have tumor enlargement during pregnancy and must be monitored closely for mass effects and hormonal changes.
- Pregnancy can be associated with complications such pituitary hemorrhage and hypophysitis.

INTRODUCTION

A normal functioning pituitary gland is vital for fertility and pregnancy. The pituitary gland undergoes significant anatomic and physiology changes during pregnancy and is required for normal fetal development. Pituitary disorders are relatively common, and any structural abnormality or hormonal dysfunction can interfere with a woman's ability to become pregnant or maintain pregnancy. In addition, pregnancy complications, such as postpartum hemorrhage and lymphocytic hypophysitis, can cause pituitary damage resulting in pituitary insufficiency, which if unrecognized can be life threatening. Pregnant women with pituitary disorders can pose complex management issues and require a multidisciplinary treatment team. This review discusses some of the more common issues that may arise when treating women with pituitary

Disclosure Statement: None.
Neuroendocrine/Pituitary Program, Division of Endocrinology, Diabetes and Metabolism, University of Florida, 1600 Southwest Archer Road, Room H2, PO Box 100226, Gainesville, FL 32610, USA
E-mail address: whitney.woodmansee@medicine.ufl.edu

Neurol Clin 37 (2019) 63–83
https://doi.org/10.1016/j.ncl.2018.09.009
0733-8619/19/© 2018 Elsevier Inc. All rights reserved.

neurologic.theclinics.com

disorders, including prepregnancy planning, pregnancy management, and post-partum care.

PITUITARY PHYSIOLOGY

The pituitary is a small gland sitting at the base of the skull that is critical for regulation of the body's hormonal systems. It has been termed the "master gland" due to its role in regulation of multiple target organs, including the thyroid, adrenal, and reproductive organs. It plays a fundamental role in the development and maintenance of pregnancy. It is divided into the anterior (adenohypophysis) and posterior (neurohypophysis) pituitary. The anterior pituitary comprises 5 main cell types: somatotropes, gonadotropes, lactotropes, thyrotropes, and corticotropes that secrete growth hormone (GH), gonadotropins (follicle-stimulating hormone [FSH], luteinizing hormone [LH]), prolactin, thyrotropin (TSH), and adrenocorticotropin (ACTH), respectively, under the control of the hypothalamus. These cells control hormonal secretion from target organs and are regulated by classic endocrine-negative feedback loops. The pituitary is involved in reproduction and lactation in women and undergoes numerous changes during pregnancy. The pituitary is known to enlarge in size during pregnancy, with largest increases noted in the first few days postpartum.[1] The normal size adult pituitary gland is approximately 5 to 10 mm in height, and during pregnancy, it can increase to 12 mm[1]; there have even been case reports of pituitary enlargement so great as to cause mass effects by applying pressure upon surrounding structures.[2] The pituitary enlargement is due to hyperplasia of the prolactin producing cells (lactotropes) and is a normal physiologic process associated with increasing prolactin levels during pregnancy. The pituitary generally returns to its baseline size within the first 6 months following delivery.[1] There are also several physiologic changes in pituitary hormonal axes during pregnancy. There are no changes in thyrotrope or corticotrope number, but there are hormonal changes in these systems. For example, TSH is frequently suppressed during the first trimester of pregnancy due to the high levels of circulating placental human chorionic gonadotropin hCG stimulating thyroid hormone production to meet increased demands during the first trimester of pregnancy.[3] Free thyroxine (T4) levels later decrease, and TSH returns to normal. Thyroid-binding globulin levels increase during pregnancy, resulting in increased total T4 and T3 (triiodothyronine). Pregnancy is associated with activation of the hypothalamic-pituitary adrenal axis as indicated by elevations in free and total cortisol levels as well as cortisol binding globulin. There are also alterations in cortisol feedback as evidenced by incomplete suppression of cortisol levels in pregnant women following dexamethasone administration.[4] In addition, there are alterations in the GH and insulin-like growth factor I (IGF-I) system as well. Pregnancy is associated with reduced somatotrope number and lower native GH levels but mildly elevated IGF-I levels, thought to be mediated by placental variant GH and IGF-I production.[5] High estrogen levels in pregnancy are thought to cause a relative GH resistance in early pregnancy that is associated with lower IGF-I levels initially. As pregnancy progresses, increasing secretion of placental variant GH causes a reduction in maternal GH and an increase in maternal IGF-I that returns to normal after delivery.[5,6] Finally, gonadotropins are suppressed as expected during pregnancy because of the high levels of circulating estrogen and progesterone.

PITUITARY ADENOMAS

Pituitary adenomas are tumors caused by monoclonal expansion of one of the main anterior pituitary cell types and are more common than one would suspect. They are the second most common brain tumor histology reported overall and are thought to account for approximately 15% to 17% of all intracranial tumors and nearly one-quarter of all benign brain tumors.[7–9] Epidemiologic studies have shown variable numbers based on the population examined, with higher prevalence rates reported in radiologic and autopsy studies due to the fact that these tumors may be clinically silent and thus underdiagnosed.[7,8] Recent studies estimate the prevalence of pituitary adenomas in the range of 78 to 94 cases/100,000 persons with an incidence of 3 to 4 cases/100,000 persons.[9,10] Pituitary tumors are more common in women compared with men and increase with age. Women tend to present earlier at a younger age with smaller tumors compared with men who present at an older age with larger tumors.[11] Pituitary tumors are described by size, with microadenomas being less than 10 mm and macroadenomas being ≥10 mm. Because they are typically benign lesions, these tumors cause symptoms by producing mass effect, by compressing surrounding brain structures, or alterations in pituitary hormonal function, either hormonal hypersecretion or hormonal deficiency. Patients can present with a wide variety of hormonal, neurologic, and psychiatric manifestations depending on the size and location of the lesion, as well as the type of hormonal system disrupted. Typical mass effect symptoms include headaches, visual loss (from compression of the optic chiasm), and cranial nerve deficits (typically cranial nerves III, IV, VI from cavernous sinus invasion). The clinical presentation also varies depending on the pituitary hormonal system that is altered and whether it is causing hormonal excess or deficiency. Reproductive dysfunction, including infertility, is a common manifestation of pituitary disease as a result of hypogonadism caused by either hyperprolactinemia or the tumor itself. Examples of hormone excess states caused by pituitary tumors include prolactinomas (prolactin tumor), acromegaly (GH tumor), Cushing disease (ACTH tumor), and TSH-producing tumors. Prolactinomas are thought to be the most common type of pituitary adenoma at approximately 40% and are more common in women than men.[7,12–14] Nonfunctioning pituitary adenomas are the second most common subtype followed by somatotrope (GH) and corticotrope (ACTH) tumors, with TSH producing tumors being very rare.[14] All patients with pituitary lesions require a detailed history and physical examination, pituitary imaging, and evaluation of pituitary hormonal status to evaluate for hormonal excess and deficiency.[12,15] Typical laboratory testing at initial presentation should include prolactin, TSH, free T4, ACTH, morning cortisol, LH, FSH, estradiol in women (E2), testosterone (T) in men, GH, and IGF-1.[12,15] Additional endocrine testing is required to diagnose hypercortisolism/Cushing disease, adrenal insufficiency, GH deficiency, and occasionally, acromegaly. Patients should also be evaluated for associated comorbidities, such as hyperglycemia/diabetes mellitus in acromegaly and Cushing disease. A general approach to the evaluation and management of pituitary adenomas is outlined in **Fig. 1** (see also reviews[12,15]). A detailed discussion of treatment options for all of the different pituitary adenoma subtypes is beyond the scope of this review, but management issues are discussed related to pregnancy in the following sections. An overview of the approach in pregnancy is reviewed in **Fig. 2**. In general, women with pituitary tumors can achieve pregnancy, although women with hypogonadism, due to either the tumor itself or hyperprolactinemia, will require assistance for conception. More women with pituitary disease are becoming pregnant due to advances in tumor and infertility treatment options. Once pregnancy is attained, all patients will require close monitoring for signs and symptoms of tumor enlargement. Patients should be monitored for mass effects and new hormonal deficiencies. Serial clinical evaluations should be performed during pregnancy with pituitary imaging done only if the patient exhibits signs or symptoms suggestive of tumor progression. Concerning symptoms include new or worsening headaches, visual changes, cranial nerve palsies, or documented new hormonal

Pituitary Adenoma/Sellar Lesion Identified
Assess for mass effects (headache, visual loss, cranial nerve palsy)
Assess pituitary hormonal function:
• Hormone excess: prolactin, GH, ACTH, TSH
• Hormone deficiency: replace as needed. Thyroid and cortisol replacement most important
Decide on treatment approach with multidisciplinary team (may require multimodal treatment)
Surgery
Medical Therapy
Observation
Early Postoperative Management:
Assess for complications:
• Neurologic status
• Endocrine function
– Diabetes insipidus
– SIADH
– Adrenal insufficiency
• Surgical patients typically evaluated 1, 6, 12 wk postoperatively.
• MRI typically repeated at 12 wk postoperatively to serve as new baseline.
Long Term Management
• Follow-up every 6 – 12 mo or as dictated by patient's clinical status.
– Hormonal assessment
– MRI (Typically annually)
• More frequent monitoring required with medical therapy and during pregnancy
• Long term assessment of hormonal status and tumor recurrence required.

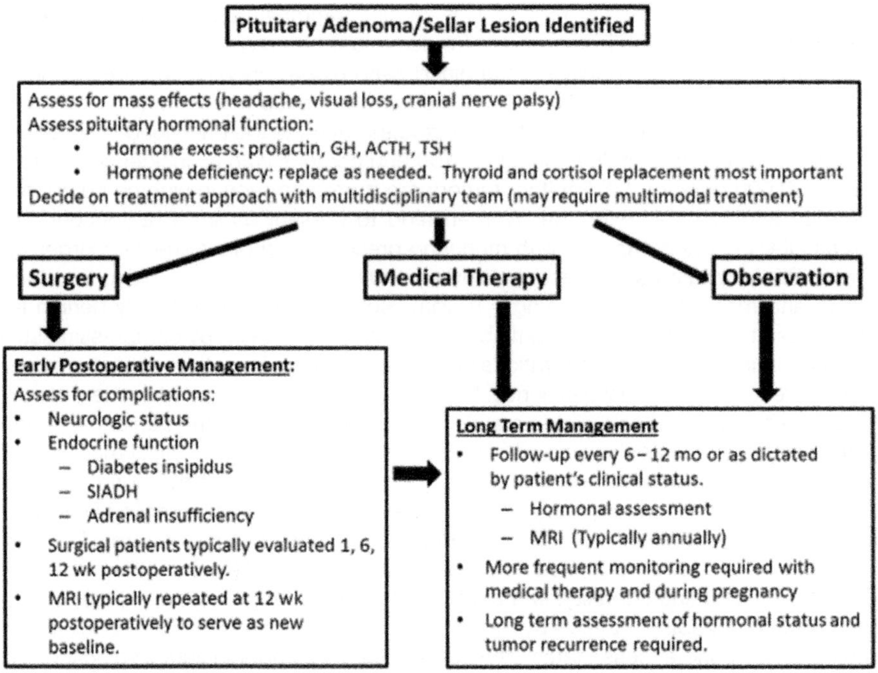

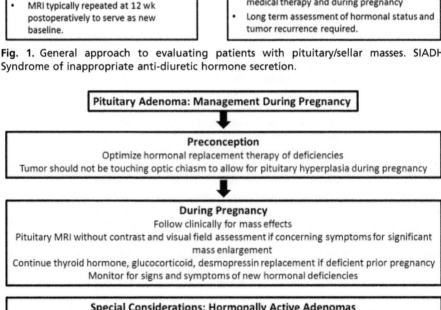

Fig. 1. General approach to evaluating patients with pituitary/sellar masses. SIADH, Syndrome of inappropriate anti-diuretic hormone secretion.

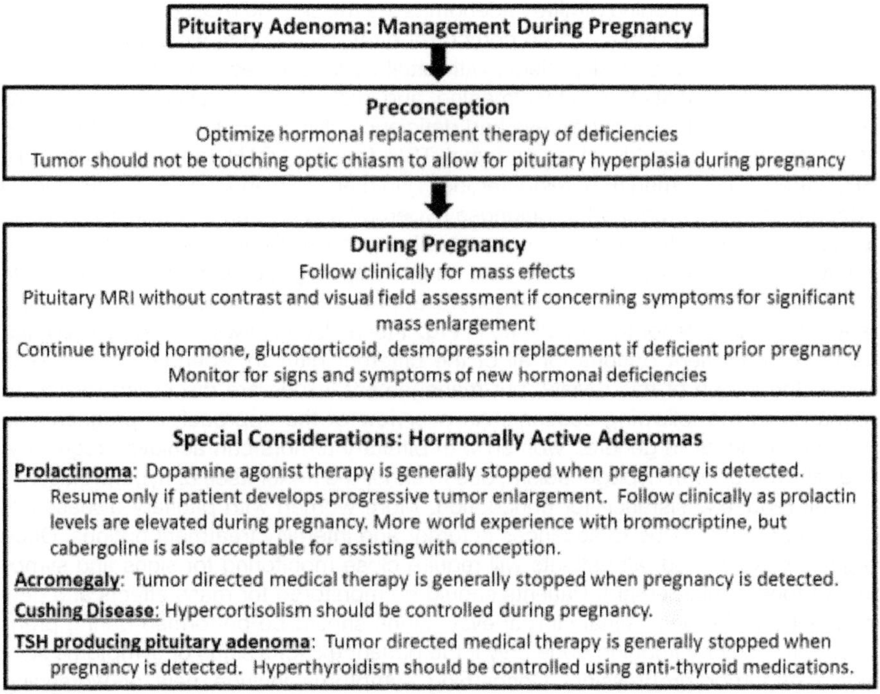

Pituitary Adenoma: Management During Pregnancy
Preconception
Optimize hormonal replacement therapy of deficiencies
Tumor should not be touching optic chiasm to allow for pituitary hyperplasia during pregnancy
During Pregnancy
Follow clinically for mass effects
Pituitary MRI without contrast and visual field assessment if concerning symptoms for significant mass enlargement
Continue thyroid hormone, glucocorticoid, desmopressin replacement if deficient prior pregnancy
Monitor for signs and symptoms of new hormonal deficiencies
Special Considerations: Hormonally Active Adenomas
Prolactinoma: Dopamine agonist therapy is generally stopped when pregnancy is detected. Resume only if patient develops progressive tumor enlargement. Follow clinically as prolactin levels are elevated during pregnancy. More world experience with bromocriptine, but cabergoline is also acceptable for assisting with conception.
Acromegaly: Tumor directed medical therapy is generally stopped when pregnancy is detected.
Cushing Disease: Hypercortisolism should be controlled during pregnancy.
TSH producing pituitary adenoma: Tumor directed medical therapy is generally stopped when pregnancy is detected. Hyperthyroidism should be controlled using anti-thyroid medications.

Fig. 2. General management of pituitary adenomas in pregnant women.

deficiencies. Some patients with functional pituitary tumors may require monitoring for worsening hormonal excess and related comorbidities (ie, Cushing disease, acromegaly). Patients with macroadenomas should have periodic formal visual field testing during pregnancy and pituitary imaging performed in cases of worsening vision. Tumor-directed medical therapy is usually discontinued in patients with functional pituitary tumors (ie, prolactinoma patients on a dopamine agonist) once pregnancy is confirmed and reinitiation of therapy considered if the patient develops symptomatic tumor growth. Most tumor-directed drugs do not have an approved indication for use in pregnancy, so appropriate counseling of the patient on potential risks and benefits is mandatory. Patients with macroadenomas at the time of conception are at higher risk of symptomatic tumor progression during pregnancy than those with microadenomas due to decreased sellar space for physiologic pituitary expansion in pregnancy. Because the pituitary enlarges during pregnancy, ideally the tumor should not be contacting the optic chiasm at the onset of pregnancy. Hypopituitarism requires close monitoring during pregnancy due to hormonal changes in pregnancy, and hormonal deficiencies, such as thyroid hormone and glucocorticoids, should be adequately replaced for optimal maternal and fetal health. Although most patients can be safely managed during pregnancy, preconception planning is desired. All patients with pituitary adenomas, irrespective of pregnancy, require long-term management and assessment of hormonal status and tumor progression.

Prolactinomas

Prolactinomas are the most common pituitary adenoma subtype and are more common in women than men.[7,12–14] They tend to be detected earlier in premenopausal women compared with postmenopausal women and men due to the presenting symptoms of galactorrhea and menstrual irregularities (amenorrhea/oligomenorrhea). Elevated prolactin levels inhibit pulsatile gonadotropin secretion and induce central hypogonadism. Some women are initially discovered during evaluation for infertility, and one series estimated that approximately 30% of women with infertility have hyperprolactinemia as a cause.[16] A more recent study found that 5.6% of asymptomatic women presenting with infertility had elevated prolactin levels and did not significantly differ from rates seen in women with irregular menses.[17] Approximately 20% of those with an elevated prolactin were found to have a pituitary microadenoma on MRI in this series.[17] Hyperprolactinemia can be due to several causes other than pituitary adenomas, so it is important to consider the differential diagnosis (such as pregnancy, hypothyroidism, and medications as other common causes) when evaluating new patients with elevated prolactin levels. Once the diagnosis of a prolactinoma is confirmed, treatment is usually recommended to control tumor growth and normalize prolactin levels for restoration of gonadal function.[13,18–20] Medical treatment with a dopamine agonist (most commonly bromocriptine or cabergoline) is the treatment of choice for most symptomatic prolactinomas, because these agents are highly effective at normalizing prolactin levels ($\sim$60%–70%), restoring gonadal function ($\sim$70%–90%) and decreasing tumor size ($\sim$60%).[19] Cabergoline is the preferred agent due to its higher efficacy and tolerability.[19] Although medical therapy alone is usually sufficient for treatment, some patients undergo surgical resection if they are resistant or intolerant of dopamine agonist therapy or for other case-specific reasons.[21,22] As with any invasive pituitary tumor, patients with invasive prolactinomas can require multimodal therapy involving surgery, medications, radiation, or a combination of treatments.[20–23] Observation with serial imaging and prolactin level monitoring may be considered for patients with asymptomatic incidental microprolactinomas.[19]

Dopamine agonist therapy is usually required for conception in women with prolactinomas, because it is often necessary to normalize prolactin levels in order to restore ovulation. Both bromocriptine and cabergoline are effective in reducing prolactin levels and restoring fertility.[19,20] Bromocriptine has historically been the drug of choice preconception, and as a result, there is more real-world experience with this drug in early pregnancy. Bromocriptine does cross the placenta, but short-term use has not been associated with increased risk of pregnancy complications or adverse fetal effects.[24–26] Very few pieces of data exist on bromocriptine use throughout gestation and its effects on the exposed infants, but it has not been associated with increased developmental abnormalities.[25] There has been less overall experience with cabergoline preconception/during early gestation, but more recent studies do not demonstrate increased risk of pregnancy complications or fetal abnormalities compared with bromocriptine or the general population.[25,27–30] A recent study examined 48 pregnancies in 33 women with macroprolactinomas who conceived on cabergoline.[31] Twenty-five women were maintained on cabergoline throughout pregnancy and did not appear to have more adverse pregnancy outcomes compared with women who had discontinued cabergoline at pregnancy confirmation.[31] Thus, cabergoline is generally regarded as an acceptable option for therapy for facilitating conception.[20,25,32] Nevertheless, clinicians generally recommend discontinuation of dopamine agonist therapy as early as possible in the pregnancy or as soon as pregnancy is confirmed if clinical status allows due to the limited experience with dopamine agonists during pregnancy and the overall desire to minimize fetal exposure to any medication.

All women with prolactinomas (and any pituitary adenoma) require close monitoring during pregnancy to detect potential tumor progression because normal pregnancy is associated with lactotrope hyperplasia, and discontinuation of dopamine agonist therapy may be associated with tumor proliferation. Most women do not have symptomatic tumor growth during pregnancy (>95%), but if a macroadenoma enlarges during pregnancy, it can cause considerable mass effects depending on its proximity to surrounding structures and may be associated with new hormonal deficiencies. The risk of tumor enlargement varies by prepregnancy tumor size. As would be expected, women with smaller tumors are at lower risk of developing symptomatic tumor enlargement (<3%) compared with women with macroadenomas.[25] Women with macroprolactinomas without prior surgery or radiation therapy are more likely (~21%) to have symptomatic enlargement than women who had previous surgery or radiation (4.7%).[25] In a recent UK study of 49 pregnancies in women with macroprolactinomas, 6 showed tumor enlargement, and none of the cases were in women previously treated with surgery or radiation.[33] Some women with macroadenomas elect surgery before pregnancy to reduce the risk of symptomatic tumor enlargement. All women should be observed for symptoms of tumor progression clinically and routinely questioned about symptoms of mass effects (ie, headaches, visual disturbances) and symptoms suggestive of new hormonal deficiencies. Serial visual field testing is recommended in women with large tumors, and new visual abnormalities or progressive headaches should be evaluated with pituitary MRI (preferably without gadolinium).[19,25] It is not recommended that prolactin levels be monitored during pregnancy because levels are physiologically elevated during pregnancy and they do not necessarily correlate with tumor activity during pregnancy.[19] Dopamine agonist therapy can be restarted if the patient develops symptomatic enlargement, and in unusual cases, surgery may be required.[19,25] Guidelines have recommended bromocriptine in this setting largely due to the greater world experience with the drug,[19] but as cabergoline use has become more common and it appears to be as safe in pregnancy, these recommendations may change. Surgery is generally the less favored option due to potential risk to the fetus, but can be performed if needed emergently or if the tumor is nonresponsive to medical therapy. Interestingly, some prolactinoma patients show improvement or resolution of hyperprolactinemia and/or tumor shrinkage following pregnancy.[34–36] There is no contraindication to breastfeeding, and it is not associated with tumor enlargement; however, patients who wish to breastfeed in the postpartum period should not restart dopamine agonists.[25]

In summary, women with prolactinomas frequently have galactorrhea, menstrual irregularities, and infertility, which can be effectively treated with dopamine agonists in order to reverse symptoms, decrease tumor size, and restore fertility. Dopamine agonists should be discontinued in most patients upon confirmation of pregnancy but can be resumed if there is evidence of tumor progression during pregnancy. Patients require close clinical monitoring during pregnancy for tumor enlargement as evidenced by new mass effect symptoms, visual field deficits, or hormonal deficiencies.

Acromegaly

Acromegaly is a rare condition caused by GH excess that is associated with multiple comorbidities and increased mortality. GH secreting pituitary adenomas are responsible for the vast majority of cases of GH excess. GH stimulates IGF-I secretion from the liver, which circulates to induce a variety of effects throughout the body. Individuals with acromegaly exhibit several somatic and metabolic changes, including soft tissue hypertrophy, osteoarthritis and changes in bone structure, organomegaly, and hyperglycemia. These changes are associated with multiple comorbidities, such as hypertension, cardiovascular disease including cardiomegaly and congestive heart failure, hyperglycemia/diabetes mellitus, colon polyps, thyroid nodules, carpal tunnel syndrome, and obstructive sleep apnea. Acromegalic patients have a 2-fold increased mortality risk compared with the general population[37] that is reversed with biochemical control of the disease.[38,39] Because these tumors are typically slow growing, symptom onset is gradual, and acromegaly is often diagnosed later in the course of the disease with larger tumors. Diagnosis is based on clinical presentation in conjunction with elevated IGF-I levels and pituitary mass on MRI. Failure to suppress GH levels in response to an oral glucose load can also be used to confirm autonomous GH secretion. Once the diagnosis has been confirmed, treatment options include surgical resection and/or medical therapy, with somatostatin analogues being the first-line medication used in patients not candidates for or not biochemically controlled with surgery.[40,41] Additional medications used to treat acromegaly include cabergoline or the GH receptor antagonist pegvisomant and are reviewed in detail in the recent consensus statement.[41] All acromegalic patients should be screened for known associated comorbidities, such as hypertension, cardiac disease, diabetes mellitus, arthritis, sleep apnea, and colon and thyroid neoplasms.[40]

Acromegaly can be difficult to diagnose during pregnancy due to placental secretion of variant GH that stimulates maternal IGF-I production, and many laboratory assays cannot reliably differentiate between the 2 forms of GH.[42] Pregnancy-specific IGF-I reference ranges are not available, further complicating the diagnosis during pregnancy. Unless diagnosis is critical, clinicians often defer diagnosis until after pregnancy. As with any woman with pituitary disease, fertility in acromegalic women is often impaired for the reasons previously discussed. Ideally, women with acromegaly are biochemically controlled with either surgery or medical therapy before attempting pregnancy. Because of the lack of long-term safety data during pregnancy, tumor-directed medical therapy (ie, somatostatin analogue, cabergoline, pegvisomant) is generally stopped when pregnancy is confirmed. Recent guidelines have suggested stopping long-acting somatostatin analogues and pegvisomant 2 months before conception and switching to the short-acting somatostatin analogue octreotide until pregnancy is confirmed.[40] This switch is not always possible in practice, but the medication should be discontinued as early as possible after conception to minimize potential risks to fetus.[40,42] Pregnant acromegalic women should be monitored closely during pregnancy for clinical disease progression, just as one would monitor women with nonfunctional pituitary tumors. Measurement of GH and IGF-I levels during pregnancy is not recommended, but patients should be assessed for headache and visual changes as symptoms of mass enlargement. Not all mass effect symptoms are due to tumor progression, and clinicians should be aware that pituitary apoplexy/hemorrhage or pituitary hyperplasia of pregnancy adjacent to residual tumor can produce symptoms. In addition, these patients should be monitored for exacerbation of known acromegalic comorbidities, such as hypertension and hyperglycemia, which can worsen when off medical therapy and during pregnancy in general. Fortunately, studies do not suggest that pregnancy accelerates GH tumor growth or worsens disease activity, and most patients show relative disease stability during pregnancy.[42–45] In fact, the relative GH resistance during pregnancy induced by high estrogen levels may help moderate IGF-I levels.[42] Medical therapy may be reinitiated with emergence of headache or visual loss. In this instance, although they are thought to be less efficacious in acromegaly than the somatostatin analogues, some clinicians may initially try the dopamine agonists, bromocriptine or cabergoline, because of a longer track record of use in pregnancy in pituitary disease. Very limited data are available for somatostatin analogue use during pregnancy at time of conception or continuously, and most use is with octreotide and not lanreotide or pasireotide. The latter 2 agents are pregnancy Food and Drug Administration class C based on animal data showing adverse fetal effects and would not be considered optimal choices for acromegalic women during pregnancy.[46,47] Low birth weight has been associated with octreotide exposure during pregnancy, but no severe fetal consequences have been reported in the small number of cases where it has been used.[42,45] A recent report of pegvisomant exposure in 35 pregnancies (27 maternal exposures and 8 paternal exposures) was published from the Pfizer global safety database.[48] These 35 pregnancies resulted in 18 live births: 14 were described as normal newborns (although 4 were premature) and 4 fetal outcomes were not reported. The remaining 17 pregnancy outcomes were as follows: 1 ectopic pregnancy, 2 miscarriages, 5 elective terminations, and 9 undetermined pregnancy outcomes. If reinitiation of medical therapy fails to address progressive mass effects, urgent surgical resection remains an option in emergent cases. Fortunately, the experience thus far in pregnant acromegalic women suggests that most do well and maintain stable disease and do not demonstrate aggressive tumor progression during pregnancy.

Cushing Disease

Cushing syndrome describes hypercortisolism due to any cause, whereas Cushing disease refers specifically to cortisol excess due to an ACTH-producing pituitary adenoma. Hypercortisolism presents clinically with central obesity, hirsutism, acne, hyperpigmented striae, infertility, easy bruising, proximal muscle weakness, cognitive dysfunction, and mood changes and is associated with several comorbidities, including hypertension, hyperglycemia, hypercoagulability, poor wound healing, impaired quality of life, and osteoporosis.[49–53] Cushing disease is associated with higher mortality rates and increased risk of cardiovascular and cerebrovascular disease.[50,54–56] Cushing disease tends to affect young women of childbearing age and is at least 3 times more prevalent in women than in men.[50] Diagnosis can be very challenging and is based on documenting endogenous hypercortisolism, determining whether cause is ACTH dependent or independent, and finally, localizing the responsible tumor (pituitary, adrenal, or ectopic source).[49,57] Once the source is identified, surgical resection is the treatment of choice.[50,57–59] Fortunately, several medical options exist for patients not cured by surgery. These options include medical therapy with steroidogenesis inhibitors (ie ketoconazole, metyrapone, mitotane [adrenolytic]), glucocorticoid antagonists (mifepristone) or pituitary directed medications, cabergoline or pasireotide.[50,57–59] Patients with Cushing disease and persistent hypercortisolism can also consider pituitary radiation or bilateral adrenalectomy. All pituitary patients require long-term observation because recurrence is not uncommon. In one series at a single institution, of 455 patients that had undergone successful transsphenoidal ACTH tumor resection, 40 required repeat surgery for recurrent Cushing disease (median time to recurrence 36 months, range 4 months to 16 years).[60]

Cushing syndrome in pregnancy exacerbates the challenges with both diagnosis and management in an already very complex disorder. First, diagnosis is complicated due to the physiologic changes in the hypothalamic pituitary adrenal axis that occur during normal pregnancy, as well as an overlap of clinical symptoms with those common in normal pregnancy, such as weight gain, striae, hypertension, and hyperglycemia. As outlined earlier, pregnancy is associated with increased total serum and urinary free cortisol during gestation, making their use for diagnosis of Cushing syndrome in pregnancy difficult.[61,62] There is some evidence that late night salivary cortisol levels may be useful for diagnosis if trimester-specific reference ranges are used.[63] Furthermore, the placenta secretes ACTH and CRH, which complicates determining whether the confirmed hypercortisolism is ACTH dependent or independent.[64] Determining whether the hypercortisolism is ACTH dependent or independent is a critical diagnostic decision point, as this directs site of imaging for tumor localization. Cushing disease is the most common cause of Cushing syndrome in nonpregnant women, whereas adrenal sources are more frequently encountered in pregnant women with confirmed hypercortisolism and account for approximately 40% to 60% of cases diagnosed in pregnancy.[61,62,65] Imaging is also more challenging in the pregnant patient due to desire to avoid exposure of the fetus to radiation associated with abdominal CT scans or gadolinium used in MRI imaging of the pituitary. Thus, abdominal ultrasound is used to image the adrenals, and pituitary MRI without gadolinium is preferred when Cushing disease is suspected. The later scenario is suboptimal because it is known that ACTH pituitary tumors are commonly very small and difficult to identify even with gadolinium administration. Treatment of hypercortisolism is recommended during pregnancy due to the adverse maternal and fetal effects of high circulating cortisol levels. A review of published cases demonstrated that women with active Cushing syndrome were more likely to have hypertension, diabetes mellitus, and preeclampsia than those with a sustained biochemical remission.[65] Other complications include those associated with active Cushing syndrome: fractures, venous thromboembolism, psychiatric symptoms, and infections. Although the fetus is partially protected from maternal hypercortisolism due to upregulation of placental 11-β hydroxysteroid dehydrogenase, which deactivates cortisol,[66] fetal demise, prematurity, intrauterine growth retardation, and adrenal insufficiency have been observed in active Cushing syndrome at higher rates than in patients in biochemical remission.[61,65] Treatment choice depends on severity of the hypercortisolism and when during the pregnancy the diagnosis is confirmed. Surgery is generally still considered the treatment of choice for Cushing syndrome and can be offered in the second trimester of pregnancy depending on case specifics. Medical management of the comorbidities of hypercortisolism (ie, hypertension, hyperglycemia) is a potential approach, particularly if symptoms are mild or the disease is detected toward the end of pregnancy. Cabergoline has been used in pituitary Cushing patients,[67,68] and as discussed in other sections of this review, it appears to be relatively safe for use in pregnancy. Finally, steroidogenesis inhibitors metyrapone and ketoconazole have been used in pregnancy, with metyrapone preferred due to potential teratogenic effects of ketoconazole.[61,69,70] Mitotane is contraindicated in pregnancy because it is an adrenolytic agent.

Cushing disease is associated with significant morbidity and mortality. Diagnosis is frequently difficult but is particularly challenging in the pregnant patient. Hypercortisolism should be treated during pregnancy if confirmed, due to the associated adverse maternal and fetal outcomes. Surgical tumor removal is preferred in many patients, but comorbidities and hypercortisolism can be medically managed if needed.

Thyrotropin-Producing Pituitary Adenomas

TSH-producing pituitary adenomas are the rarest of all the pituitary tumors at less than 1%, with an estimated prevalence of approximately 2.8 cases per million.[71] Patients present with elevated peripheral thyroid hormones (T4 and T3), a nonsuppressed TSH, and signs and symptoms of hyperthyroidism. Diagnosis is confirmed by demonstrating a pituitary adenoma on MRI and dynamic testing of the hypothalamic pituitary thyroid axis to assist with distinguishing from another rare genetic condition known as resistance to thyroid hormone. Autonomous TSH secretion is documented by performing stimulatory and inhibitory testing of the axis. Patients will TSH-producing pituitary tumors will show a blunted TSH response to thyrotropin-releasing hormone and will fail to suppress TSH in response to T3 administration.[72–74] Alpha subunit (TRH is a heterodimer of TSHβ and α subunits) levels are often elevated. The treatment of choice is pituitary tumor removal[72,73] as it is generally very effective at controlling hormonal hypersecretion.[75] If surgery does not successfully remove the entire tumor or the patient is not a surgical candidate, somatostatin analogues have shown efficacy in causing tumor shrinkage and reduction in TSH secretion with restoration of euthyroidism.[72,73,75] Sometimes antithyroid medications such as methimazole are added to normalize thyroid function. Given that this is such a rare tumor, there is a paucity of data regarding pregnancy related outcomes in women with TSH-producing pituitary tumors. The same general principles apply when managing these patients as other hormonally active tumor patients. If the patient is on a somatostatin analogue preconception, then it is stopped prepregnancy if possible and not continued during pregnancy unless there is evidence of disease progression. Euthyroidism is very important for maternal and fetal outcomes, and normal thyroid function is critical preconception and during pregnancy.[76] Antithyroid medications can be used during pregnancy to treat the hyperthyroidism caused by the TSH-producing tumor if needed.

HYPOPITUITARISM

Hypopituitarism occurs when there is partial or total loss of pituitary function and more commonly involves anterior pituitary dysfunction (see reviews[77,78]). Hypopituitarism can be congenital or acquired. Acquired causes are typically due to structural lesions involving the sellar/suprasellar region or its related treatment, such as surgery or radiation. Pituitary insufficiency caused by surgery is related to tumor size and location as well as experience of the neurosurgeon. A recent series of 80 patients who underwent endoscopic transsphenoidal pituitary surgery in a high-volume pituitary center by an experienced surgeon demonstrated only a 6.3% incidence of increased pituitary deficiency from preoperative baseline.[79] Other causes include infiltrative/inflammatory, infectious, vascular, or traumatic pituitary disorders. Medications can cause functional or chronic pituitary insufficiency. Examples include opiate-induced hypogonadism and adrenal insufficiency,[80,81] and immune checkpoint inhibitor-induced hypophysitis resulting in hypopituitarism (ie, anti-CTLA-4 and anti-PD-1 used in malignancies such as malignant melanoma).[82] Depending on the cause and hormone system affected, hypopituitarism can present insidiously with chronic subtle symptoms or acutely with life-threatening symptoms, as in adrenal crisis. Any combination of hormonal deficiencies is possible, and patients present with symptoms that vary based on which target organ hormone is missing. Diagnosis is based on clinical history, examination, and laboratory results demonstrating deficiency. Each hormonal axis should be assessed, and the laboratory tests are as outlined earlier in the discussion of the evaluation of a sellar/suprasellar mass. ACTH and GH deficiency often require stimulation testing to confirm the deficiency. Posterior pituitary dysfunction is associated with deficiency of arginine vasopressin (antidiuretic hormone) and causes central diabetes insipidus. The symptoms of diabetes insipidus are related to inability to concentrate urine due to vasopressin deficiency and include polyuria, polydipsia, and hypernatremia if water access is limited. A water deprivation test can be performed to confirm the diagnosis.

Hypopituitarism treatment involves replacing the deficient target organ hormones. Fortunately, all of the target endocrine hormones can be replaced with the exception of prolactin. The Endocrine Society has published guidelines in 2016 outlining recommendations for optimal hormonal replacement in hypopituitarism,[78] including pregnant patients, which are briefly summarized in **Table 1**.

The pregnant woman with hypopituitarism should continue most hormonal replacement therapy during pregnancy. Thyroid hormone and adrenal insufficiency must be treated during pregnancy for optimal fetal development and health of the mother. Adrenal insufficiency should be treated with replacement glucocorticoids, with hydrocortisone being the preferred formulation. Hydrocortisone is preferred in part due to the fact it is metabolized by placental 11-β hydroxysteroid dehydrogenase, thus protecting the fetus from excess exposure.[66] As in the nonpregnant patient, hydrocortisone dosing is generally 15-20 mg total per day in divided doses and is based on clinical status. Generally, pregnant women do not require increased glucocorticoid replacement doses in early pregnancy but may require higher doses as pregnancy progresses.[66] Hydrocortisone stress dosing is required during illness and at the time of delivery. Mineralocorticoid replacement is not needed in patients with central adrenal insufficiency due to the intact aldosterone system. Thyroid hormone replacement should also be continued during pregnancy with a goal to maintain free or total T4 levels within the normal range. Many free T4 assays are not as accurate in pregnancy due to an increase in thyroxine binding globulin and relative decrease in albumin; thus, some advocate monitoring total T4 levels during pregnancy and adjusting up the reference range by 50% if method and pregnancy trimester-specific reference ranges for free T4 are not available.[76] Because central hypothyroidism is due to TSH deficiency, TSH cannot be used reliably to guide therapy. It should also be recognized that the demand for thyroid hormone increases during pregnancy and that many women with hypothyroidism require an increase in their levothyroxine dose during pregnancy.[83] Women should be advised to alert the clinician as soon as pregnancy is confirmed so thyroid hormone levels can be checked and levothyroxine doses adjusted as needed. Thyroid status should be monitored closely during pregnancy. Normal thyroid function is desired during pregnancy because inadequately treated hypothyroidism has been associated with adverse pregnancy outcomes and fetal neurocognitive development.[76] Women with central diabetes insipidus should continue desmopressin (DDAVP) replacement therapy during pregnancy and doses

Table 1
Summary of evaluation and management of hypopituitarism

Hormonal Deficiency	Target Organ	Clinical Presentation	Diagnosis	Treatment	Monitoring
ACTH	Adrenal	Nausea, vomiting dizziness, fatigue, hypotension, abnormal electrolytes	Low cortisol ACTH stimulation test	GCC hydrocortisone preferred	Clinical status, avoid over-replacement
TSH	Thyroid	Weight gain, fatigue, constipation, hair loss, cold intolerance, cognitive dysfunction	Low free or total T4 with normal/low TSH	Levothyroxine	Clinical response, free or total T4 levels, cannot use TSH
FSH/LH	Gonad	Infertility Women (W): Menstrual irregularities Men (M): Erectile dysfunction	Low estradiol (W) or testosterone (M) with normal/low FSH/LH	Consider HRT: premenopausal W: Estrogen/progesterone M: Testosterone	Clinical response, W: Menses, M: Erectile function, PSA, prostate examination, Hct, T levels
GH	Liver	Central obesity, fatigue, impaired QOL	Low IGF-I GH stimulation test	GH	Clinical response IGF-I levels
Prolactin	Breast	Inability to lactate	Low prolactin	None	None
AVP	Kidney	Polyuria, polydipsia, inability to concentrate urine	Water deprivation test	DDAVP	Clinical response, urine output, electrolytes

Abbreviations: AVP, arginine vasopressin; GCC, glucocorticoids; Hct, hematocrit; HRT, hormone replacement therapy; PSA, prostate-specific antigen; QOL, quality of life.

should be adjusted to control symptoms of polyuria and polydipsia and maintain normal electrolyte levels. DDAVP dose requirements may also increase during pregnancy due to the action of placental vasopressinase, which degrades arginine vasopressin.[84] Adult GH deficiency is associated with central adiposity, fatigue, impaired quality of life, and unfavorable lipid profiles, and many patients receive long-term GH replacement therapy.[85,86] Although there are very few data concerning the continued use of GH during pregnancy,[87] studies have demonstrated successful pregnancies can be achieved without replacement.[88] It generally is recommended that GH therapy be discontinued during pregnancy because data regarding safety in pregnancy are lacking[78] and the placenta does make a variant GH that regulates maternal IGF-I during pregnancy.[89,90]

Finally, infertility is frequently encountered in women with pituitary insufficiency and universal in women with central hypogonadism. All women with central hypogonadism and many women with other hormonal deficiencies will require reproductive assistance. Optimal thyroid and glucocorticoid replacement is also important for fertility in women with hypopituitarism.

Sheehan Syndrome

Sheehan syndrome is an uncommon complication of postpartum hemorrhage resulting in pituitary infarction/necrosis. Pituitary apoplexy refers specifically to the acute syndrome of sudden hemorrhagic pituitary infarction associated with rapid onset of symptoms (headache, visual loss, and pituitary insufficiency) and usually occurs in the setting of a pituitary adenoma. Although Sheehan syndrome can present with acute pituitary hemorrhage or sudden apoplexy, it is more frequently delayed in its clinical presentation. It is more common in geographic areas with less access to medical care due to the higher rates of postpartum hemorrhage observed. It has typically been thought to be caused by ischemia and infarction of the pituitary gland due to hypovolemia and the resulting hypotension that occurs with significant blood loss or hemorrhagic shock in postpartum hemorrhage.[91,92] Others have also postulated a potential role for thrombosis (due to the hypercoagulability of pregnancy) and vasospasm.[92–94] Autoimmunity has also been thought to play a role in the syndrome,[95,96] although in a recent prospective study of 20 women with postpartum hemorrhage and variable pituitary hormonal deficiencies, none of the women had positive antipituitary antibodies.[97] Interestingly, the ensuing hypopituitarism following postpartum hemorrhage can be acute or delayed,[98,99] and pituitary function can recover over time.[97] As with any cause of hypopituitarism, symptoms can range from life threatening to very mild and nonspecific, such as fatigue and weakness depending on the acuity of the deficiency and which hormonal axis is affected. One retrospective study of 114 patients with Sheehan syndrome documented an average delay of 19.7 years after pregnancy to attain the diagnosis.[99] Eighty-five percent of these patients with Sheehan syndrome had amenorrhea immediately after delivery, and 42% of patients had agalactia after delivery, which can be symptoms to clue the provider in to a possible diagnosis of Sheehan syndrome.[99] Panhypopituitarism was identified in 55.3% of patients, and the remaining 44.7% had partial hypopituitarism, all of whom had GH and gonadotropin deficiency. Some patients demonstrated progressive loss of pituitary function over time, and no patient had recovery of pituitary function.[99] Small sella size appeared to be a risk factor for Sheehan syndrome in this study. In another recent prospective study of 20 women with postpartum hemorrhage, 95% had one pituitary hormonal deficiency detected at 4 weeks postpartum and 60% had 2 or more hormonal deficiencies, with GH and cortisol axis being the most frequent.[97] These patients were reevaluated 24 to 28 weeks postpartum, and although many showed recovery of pituitary function, 5 out of 20 (25%) had cortisol and GH deficiency.[97] GH deficiency was noted in greater than 50% (11/20) at the second evaluation.[97]

Sheehan syndrome is fortunately relatively uncommon, particularly in communities with low rates of postpartum hemorrhage. Nevertheless, the clinician should be alerted to the possibility of pituitary necrosis and insufficiency in any woman who suffers postpartum hemorrhage. Presentation can be acute or more commonly delayed when women present with subtle, nonspecific symptoms. Pituitary hormonal deficiency can be partial or complete, and treatment is aimed at restoring the specific target organ deficiency as with any cause of hypopituitarism.

Lymphocytic Hypophysitis

Hypophysitis is the term used to describe inflammation of the pituitary gland, which can result in enlargement of the gland and cause mass effects and pituitary hormonal insufficiency. It can be categorized by cause (primary or secondary), histologic type (lymphocytic, granulomatous, xanthomatous, or plasmacytic), and involved portion of the gland (anterior, posterior, or infundibulum).[100] Lymphocytic hypophysitis is the most common histologic subtype. It is an autoimmune-mediated disorder that affects approximately 3-fold more women than men and is associated with pregnancy.[100–102] Lymphocytic hypophysitis can involve infiltration of the infundibulum, anterior pituitary, and/or posterior pituitary with lymphocytes.[100–102] Patients typically present during pregnancy (usually third trimester) or postpartum with a wide range of symptoms, which depend on the degree of pituitary enlargement from inflammation and ensuing mass effect or hormonal deficiency. Mass effects, including headaches and visual symptoms, are not uncommon, and anterior pituitary insufficiency is expected, with diabetes insipidus being less common.[100–103] Multiple hormonal deficiencies are found in most cases, with thyroid hormone and cortisol deficiency being very common.[100,103,104]

Diagnosis involves laboratory evaluation of pituitary function and pituitary imaging. Because of the temporal relationship with pregnancy, it can be difficult to distinguish clinically between lymphocytic hypophysitis and Sheehan syndrome. MRI characteristics can be helpful because the pituitary affected by lymphocytic hypophysitis is often symmetrically enlarged with homogenous enhancement by gadolinium and

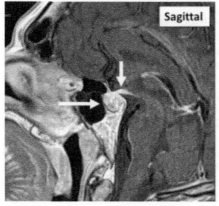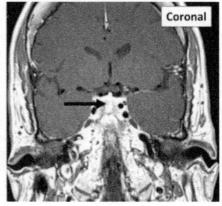

Fig. 3. Representative MRI of a patient with lymphocytic hypophysitis showing diffuse pituitary enlargement (*horizontal arrows*) and pituitary infundibulum thickening (*vertical arrow*).

pituitary stalk thickening (an example is shown in **Fig. 3**). When the neurohypophysis is affected, there can be loss in intrinsic T1 hyperintensity.[103] A recent article has also correlated more specific MRI findings in autoimmune hypophysitis with type of hormonal deficiency.[105] Anti-pituitary and anti-hypothalamic antibodies can be positive in this condition and support the diagnosis.[106] Diagnosis can be confirmed by pituitary biopsy, but this is not consistently performed for diagnosis due to the invasive nature of the procedure. Tissue confirmation would certainly be obtained in patients requiring neurosurgical decompression for mass effect symptoms.

Current treatment of lymphocytic hypophysitis is generally symptomatic, and clinicians have tried several different approaches, including conservative management, high-dose glucocorticoid therapy, and other immunosuppressive medications, such as azathioprine, neurosurgical resection, and radiation. Although there has not been a standardized approach, observation or high-dose steroids are used more initially, and more aggressive treatments, such as surgery or radiation, are reserved for large lesions with mass effects/visual loss or progressive cases. Previously it has not been clear whether glucocorticoids were superior to supportive care alone, but in a recent study of 20 patients with autoimmune hypophysitis, treatment with 50 mg oral prednisone daily was associated with significant improvement in hypophysitis and pituitary function compared with conservative management alone.[107] Other studies have shown stabilization or improvement with observation/supportive care alone.[108] It remains to be seen whether high-dose glucocorticoid will become the initial treatment of choice, and currently, an individualized approach is best according to the specific patient presentation. Hormonal deficiencies should be corrected as appropriate.

SUMMARY

The pituitary controls a wide range of physiologic systems and affects every organ in the body. Normal pituitary function is required for fertility and optimal health. Pituitary disorders are relatively common, particularly pituitary adenomas. Patients with pituitary adenoma require full evaluation for tumor mass effects and hormonal alterations, either hyperfunction or hypofunction. Treatment of choice depends on the type of pituitary tumor and whether it is hormonally active. Medical therapy is preferred in prolactin-producing tumors, whereas neurosurgical resection is preferred in most other functional and nonfunctional pituitary adenomas. Because of advancements in the care of pituitary patients and improvement in fertility induction, more women with pituitary tumors are becoming pregnant. With close monitoring and management of hormonal deficiencies or excesses, most women with pituitary disorders can have successful pregnancies.

REFERENCES

1. Dinc H, Esen F, Demirici A, et al. Pituitary dimensions and volume measurements in pregnancy and post-partum. MR assessment. Acta Radiol 1998;39:64–9.

2. Inoue T, Hotta A, Awai M, et al. Loss of vision due to a physiologic pituitary enlargement during normal pregnancy. Graefes Arch Clin Exp Ophthalmol 2007;245(7):1049–51.

3. Moleti M, Trimarchi F, Vermiglio F. Thyroid physiology in pregnancy. Endocr Pract 2014;20(6):589–96.

4. Lindsay JR, Nieman LK. The hypothalamic–pituitary–adrenal axis in pregnancy: challenges in disease detection and treatment. Endocr Rev 2005;26:775–99.

5. Karaca Z, Tanriverdi F, Unluhizarci K, et al. Pregnancy and pituitary disorders. Eur J Endocrinol 2010;162(3):453–75.
6. Wu Z, Bidlingmaier M, Friess SC, et al. A new nonisotopic, highly sensitive assay for the measurement of human placental growth hormone: development and clinical implications. J Clin Endocrinol Metab 2003;88(2):804–11.
7. Ezzat S, Asa SL, Couldwell WT, et al. The prevalence of pituitary adenomas: a systematic review. Cancer 2004;101(3):613–9.
8. Aflorei ED, Korbonits M. Epidemiology and etiopathogenesis of pituitary adenomas. J Neurooncol 2014;117:379–94.
9. Ostrom QT, Gittleman H, Xu J, et al. CBTRUS statistical report: primary brain and other central nervous system tumors diagnosed in the United States in 2009-2013. Neuro Oncol 2016;18(suppl 5):v1–75.
10. Karavitaki N. Prevalence and incidence of pituitary adenomas. Ann Endocrinol (Paris) 2012;73(2):79–80.
11. McDowell BD, Wallace RB, Carnahan RM, et al. Demographic differences in incidence for pituitary adenoma. Pituitary 2011;14(1):23–30.
12. Freda PU, Beckers AM, Katznelson L, et al, Endocrine Society. Pituitary incidentaloma: an endocrine society clinical practice guideline. J Clin Endocrinol Metab 2011;96(4):894–904.
13. Casaneuva FF, Molitch ME, Schlechte JA, et al. Guidelines of the pituitary society for the diagnosis and management of prolactinomas. Clin Endocrinol (Oxf) 2006;65(2):265–73.
14. Fernandez A, Karavitaki N, Wass JA. Prevalence of pituitary adenomas: a community-based, cross-sectional study in Banbury (Oxfordshire, UK). Clin Endocrinol (Oxf) 2010;72(3):377–82.
15. Woodmansee WW, Carmichael J, Kelly D, et al. American Association of Clinical Endocrinologists and American College of Endocrinology Disease state clinical review: postoperative management following pituitary surgery. Endocr Pract 2015;21(7):832–8.
16. Molitch ME, Reichlin S. Hyperprolactinemic disorders. Dis Mon 1982;28(9): 1–58.
17. Souter I, Baltagi LM, Toth TL, et al. Prevalence of hyperprolactinemia and abnormal magnetic resonance imaging findings in a population with infertility. Fertil Steril 2010;94(3):1159–62.
18. Klibanski A. Prolactinomas. N Engl J Med 2010;362:1219–26.
19. Melmed S, Casanueva FF, Hoffman AR, et al. Diagnosis and treatment of hyperprolactinemia: an endocrine society clinical practice guideline. J Clin Endocrinol Metab 2011;96(2):273–88.
20. Wong A, Eloy JA, Couldwell WT, et al. Update on prolactinomas. Part 2: treatment and management strategies. J Clin Neurosci 2015;22:1568–74.
21. Molitch ME. Pharmacologic resistance in prolactinoma patients. Pituitary 2005; 8:43–52.
22. Smith TR, Hulou MM, Huang KT, et al. Current indications for the surgical treatment of prolactinomas. J Clin Neurosci 2015;22:1785–91.
23. Vilar L, Abucham J, Albuquerque JL, et al. Controversial issues in the management of hyperprolactinemia and prolactinomas - An overview by the Neuroendocrinology Department of the Brazilian Society of Endocrinology and Metabolism. Arch Endocrinol Metab 2018;62(2):236–63.
24. Molitch ME. Prolactinoma in pregnancy. Best Pract Res Clin Endocrinol Metab 2011;25(6):885–96.

25. Molitch ME. Endocrinology in pregnancy: management of the pregnant patient with a prolactinoma. Eur J Endocrinol 2015;172(5):R205–13.
26. Raymond JP, Goldstein E, Konopka P, et al. Follow-up of children born of bromocriptine-treated mothers. Horm Res 1985;22:239–46.
27. Lebbe M, Hubinont C, Bernard P, et al. Outcome of 100 pregnancies initiated under treatment with cabergoline in hyperprolactinaemic women. Clin Endocrinol (Oxf) 2010;73(2):236–42.
28. Stalldecker G, Mallea-Gil MS, Guitelman M, et al. Effects of cabergoline on pregnancy and embryo-fetal development: retrospective study on 103 pregnancies and a review of the literature. Pituitary 2010;13(4):345–50.
29. Glezer A, Bronstein MD. Prolactinomas, cabergoline and pregnancy. Endocrine 2014;47(1):64–9.
30. Arauju B, Belo S, Carvalho D. Pregnancy and tumor outcomes in women with prolactinoma. Exp Clin Endocrinol Diabetes 2017;125(10):642–8.
31. Rastogi A, Bhadada SK, Bhansali A. Pregnancy and tumor outcomes in infertile women with macroprolactinoma on cabergoline therapy. Gynecol Endocrinol 2017;33(4):270–3.
32. Maiter D. Prolactinoma and pregnancy: from the wish of conception to lactation. Ann Endocrinol (Paris) 2016;77(2):128–34.
33. Lambert K, Rees K, Seed PT, et al. Macroprolactinomas and nonfunctioning pituitary adenomas and pregnancy outcomes. Obstet Gynecol 2017;129(1):185–94.
34. Crosignani PG, Mattei AM, Severini V, et al. Long-term effects of time, medical treatment and pregnancy in 176 hyperprolactinemic women. Eur J Obstet Gynecol Reprod Biol 1992;44(3):175–80.
35. Badawy SZ, Marziale JC, Rosenbaum AE, et al. The long-term effects of pregnancy and bromocriptine treatment on prolactinomas–the value of radiologic studies. Early Pregnancy 1997;3(4):306–11.
36. Domingue ME, Devuyst F, Alexopoulou O, et al. Outcome of prolactinoma after pregnancy and lactation: a study on 73 patients. Clin Endocrinol (Oxf) 2014;80(5):642–8.
37. Orme SM, McNally RJ, Cartwright RA, et al. Mortality and cancer incidence in acromegaly: a retrospective cohort study. United Kingdom Acromegaly Study Group. J Clin Endocrinol Metab 1998;83(8):2730–4.
38. Holdaway IM, Bolland MJ, Gamble GD. A meta-analysis of the effect of lowering serum levels of GH and IGF-I on mortality in acromegaly. Eur J Endocrinol 2008;159:89–95.
39. Dekkers OM, Biermasz NR, Pereira AM, et al. Mortality in acromegaly: a meta-analysis. J Clin Endocrinol Metab 2008;93:61–7.
40. Katznelson L, Laws ER Jr, Melmed S, et al, Endocrine Society. Acromegaly: an endocrine society clinical practice guideline. J Clin Endocrinol Metab 2014;99(11):3933–51.
41. Melmed S, Bronstein MD, Chanson P, et al. A consensus statement on acromegaly therapeutic outcomes. Nat Rev Endocrinol 2018;14(9):552–61.
42. Abucham J, Bronstein MD, Dias ML. Management of endocrine disease: acromegaly and pregnancy: a contemporary review. Eur J Endocrinol 2017;177(1):R1–12.
43. Caron P, Broussaud S, Bertherat J, et al. Acromegaly and pregnancy: a retrospective multicenter study of 59 pregnancies in 46 women. J Clin Endocrinol Metab 2010;95(10):4680–7.

44. Cheng S, Grasso L, Martinez-Orozco JA, et al. Pregnancy in acromegaly: experience from two referral centers and systematic review of the literature. Clin Endocrinol (Oxf) 2012;76(2):264–71.

45. Cheng V, Faiman C, Kennedy L, et al. Pregnancy and acromegaly: a review. Pituitary 2012;15(1):59–63.

46. Somatuline Depot (lanreotide) [package insert]. Signes, France: Ipsen Pharma Biotech; 2014.

47. Signifor (pasireotide) [package insert]. Stein, Switzerland: Novartis Pharma Stein AG; 2012.

48. van der Lely AJ, Gomez R, Heissler JF, et al. Pregnancy in acromegaly patients treated with pegvisomant. Endocrine 2015;49(3):769–73.

49. Nieman LK, Biller BM, Findling JW, et al. The diagnosis of Cushing's syndrome: an endocrine society clinical practice guideline. J Clin Endocrinol Metab 2008; 93(5):1526–40.

50. Pivonello R, De Leo M, Cozzolino A, et al. The treatment of Cushing's disease. Endocr Rev 2015;36(4):385–486.

51. Sharma ST, Nieman LK, Feelders RA. Comorbidities in Cushing's disease. Pituitary 2015;18:188–94.

52. Coelho MCA, Santos CV, Neto LV, et al. Adverse effects of glucocorticoids: coagulopathy. Eur J Endocrinol 2015;173:M11–21.

53. Santos A, Crespo I, Aulinas A, et al. Quality of life in Cushing's syndrome. Pituitary 2015;18(2):195–200.

54. Webb SM, Mo D, Lamberts SW, et al, International HypoCCS Advisory Board. Metabolic, cardiovascular, and cerebrovascular outcomes in growth hormone-deficient subjects with previous Cushing's disease or non-functioning pituitary adenoma. J Clin Endocrinol Metab 2010;95(2):630–8.

55. Dekkers OM, Biermasz NR, Pereira AM, et al. Mortality in patients treated for Cushing's disease is increased, compared with patients treated for nonfunctioning pituitary macroadenoma. J Clin Endocrinol Metab 2007;92(3):976–81.

56. Van Haalen FM, Broersen LH, Jorgensen JO, et al. Management of endocrine disease: mortality remains increased in Cushing's disease despite biochemical remission: a systematic review and meta-analysis. Eur J Endocrinol 2015; 172(4):R143–9.

57. Loriaux DL. Diagnosis and differential diagnosis of Cushing's syndrome. N Engl J Med 2017;376(15):1451–9.

58. Nieman LK. Update in the medical therapy of Cushing's disease. Curr Opin Endocrinol Diabetes Obes 2013;20(4):330–4.

59. Nieman LK, Biller BM, Findling JW, et al. Treatment of Cushing's syndrome: an endocrine society clinical practice guideline. J Clin Endocrinol Metab 2015; 100(8):2807–31.

60. Patil CG, Veeravagu A, Prevedello DM, et al. Outcomes after repeat transsphenoidal surgery for recurrent Cushing's disease. Neurosurgery 2008;63(2): 266–70.

61. Bronstein MD, Machado MC, Fragoso MC. Management of endocrine disease. Management of pregnancy patients with Cushing's syndrome. Eur J Endocrinol 2015;173:R85–91.

62. Brue T, Amodru V, Castinetti F. Management of endocrine disease. Management of Cushing's syndrome during pregnancy: solved and unsolved questions. Eur J Endocrinol 2018;178:R259–66.

63. Lopes LM, Francisco RP, Galletta MA, et al. Determination of nighttime salivary cortisol during pregnancy: comparison with values in non-pregnancy and Cushing's disease. Pituitary 2016;19:30–8.

64. Lindsay JR, Jonklaas J, Oldfield EH, et al. Cushing's syndrome during pregnancy: personal experience and review of the literature. J Clin Endocrinol Metab 2005;90:3077–83.

65. Caimari F, Valassi E, Garbayo P, et al. Cushing's syndrome and pregnancy outcomes: a systematic review of published cases. Endocrine 2017;55:555–63.

66. Langlois F, Lim DST, Fleseriu M. Update on adrenal insufficiency: diagnosis and management in pregnancy. Curr Opin Endocrinol Diabetes Obes 2017;24: 184–92.

67. Nakhleh A, Saiegh L, Reut M, et al. Cabergoline treatment for recurrent Cushing's disease during pregnancy. Hormones (Athens) 2016;15(3):453–8.

68. Woo I, Ehsanipoor RM. Cabergoline therapy for Cushing's disease throughout pregnancy. Obstet Gynecol 2013;122(2 Pt 2):485–7.

69. Lim WH, Torpy DJ, Jeffries WS. The medical management of Cushing's syndrome during pregnancy. Eur J Obstet Gynecol Reprod Biol 2013;168:1–6.

70. Biller BM, Grossman AB, Stewart PM, et al. Treatment of adrenocorticotropin dependent Cushing's syndrome: a consensus statement. J Clin Endocrinol Metab 2008;93:2454–62.

71. Onnestam L, Berinder K, Burman P, et al. National incidence and prevalence of TSH-secreting pituitary adenomas in Sweden. J Clin Endocrinol Metab 2013;98: 626–35.

72. Beck-Peccoz P, Persani L, Mannavola D, et al. TSH-secreting adenomas. Best Pract Res Clin Endocrinol Metab 2009;23:597–606.

73. Beck-Peccoz P, Lania A, Beckers A, et al. European thyroid association guidelines for the diagnosis and treatment of thyrotropin-secreting pituitary. Eur Thyroid J 2013;2:76–82.

74. Tjörnstrand A, Nyström HF. Diagnosis of endocrine disease. Diagnostic approach to TSH-producing pituitary adenoma. Eur J Endocrinol 2017;177: R183–97.

75. Malchiodi E, Profka E, Ferrante E, et al. Thyrotropin-secreting pituitary adenomas: outcome of pituitary surgery and irradiation. J Clin Endocrinol Metab 2014;99(6):2069–76.

76. Alexander EK, Pearce EN, Brent GA, et al. 2017 guidelines of the American Thyroid Association for the diagnosis and management of thyroid disease during pregnancy and postpartum. Thyroid 2017;27(3):315–89.

77. Kim SY. Diagnosis and treatment of hypopituitarism. Endocrinol Metab (Seoul) 2015;30(4):443–55.

78. Fleseriu M, Hashim IA, Karavitaki N, et al. Hormonal replacement in hypopituitarism in adults: an Endocrine Society Clinical Practice Guideline. J Clin Endocrinol Metab 2016;101(11):3888–921.

79. Laws ER, Iuliano SL, Cote DJ, et al. A benchmark for preservation of normal pituitary function after endoscopic transsphenoidal surgery for pituitary macroadenomas. World Neurosurg 2016;91:371–5.

80. Gudin JA, Laitman A, Najamachu S. Opioid related endocrinopathy. Pain Med 2015;16(Suppl 1):S9–15.

81. Donegan D, Bancos I. Opioid-induced adrenal insufficiency. Mayo Clin Proc 2018;93(7):937–44.

82. Joshi MN, Whitelaw BC, Palomar MT, et al. Immune checkpoint inhibitor-related hypophysitis and endocrine dysfunction: clinical review. Clin Endocrinol (Oxf) 2016;85(3):331–9.

83. Alexander EK, Marqusee E, Lawrence J, et al. Timing and magnitude of increases in levothyroxine requirements during pregnancy in women with hypothyroidism. N Engl J Med 2004;351:241–9.

84. Durr JA, Lindheimer MD. Diagnosis and management of diabetes insipidus during pregnancy. Endocr Pract 1996;2:353–61.

85. Molitch ME, Clemmons DR, Malozowski S, et al, Endocrine Society. Evaluation and treatment of adult growth hormone deficiency: an Endocrine Society clinical practice guideline. J Clin Endocrinol Metab 2011;96(6):1587–609.

86. Jorgensen JOL, Juul A. Therapy of endocrine disease: growth hormone replacement therapy in adults: 30 years of personal clinical experience. Eur J Endocrinol 2018;179(1):R47–56.

87. Wiren L, Boguszewski CL, Johannsson G. Growth hormone (GH) replacement therapy in GH-deficient women during pregnancy. Clin Endocrinol 2002;57(2):235–9.

88. Curran AJ, Peacey SR, Shalet S. Is maternal growth hormone essential for a normal pregnancy? Eur J Endocrinol 1998;139:54–8.

89. Caufriez A, Frankenne F, Hennen G, et al. Regulation of maternal IGF-I by placental GH in normal and abnormal pregnancies. Am J Physiol Endocrinol Metab 1993;265:E572–7.

90. Lonberg U, Damm P, Anderson A-M, et al. Increase in maternal placental growth hormone during pregnancy and disappearance during parturition in normal and growth hormone deficient pregnancies. Am J Obstet Gynecol 2003;188(1):247–51.

91. Karaca Z, Laway BA, Dokmetas HS, et al. Sheehan syndrome. Nat Rev Dis Primers 2016;2:16092.

92. Dahan MH, Tan SL. A primer on pituitary injury for the obstetrician gynecologist: Simmond's disease, Sheehan's syndrome, traumatic injury, Dahan's syndrome, pituitary apopolexy and lymphocytic hypophysitis. Minerva Ginecologica 2017;69(2):190–4.

93. Gokalp D, Tuzcu A, Bahceci M, et al. Analysis of thrombophilic genetic mutations in patients with Sheehan's syndrome: is thrombophilia responsible for the pathogenesis of Sheehan's syndrome? Pituitary 2011;14:168–73.

94. Kuriya A, Morris DV, Dahan MH. Pituitary injury and persistent hypofunction resulting from a peripartum non-hemorrhagic, vaso-occlusive event. Endocrinol Diabetes Metab Case Rep 2015;2015:150001.

95. Goswami R, Kochupillai N, Crock PA, et al. Pituitary autoimmunity in patients with Sheehan's syndrome. J Clin Endocrinol Metab 2002;87:4137–41.

96. Atmaca H, Arasli M, Yazici ZA, et al. Lymphocyte subpopulations in Sheehan's syndrome. Pituitary 2013;16(2):202–7.

97. González-González JG, Borjas-Almaguer OD, Salcido-Montenegro A, et al. Sheehan's syndrome revisited: underlying autoimmunity or hypoperfusion? Int J Endocrinol 2018;2018:8415860.

98. Matsuzaki S, Endo M, Ueda Y, et al. A case of acute Sheehan's syndrome and literature review: a rare but life-threatening complication of postpartum hemorrhage. BMC Pregnancy Childbirth 2017;17(1):188.

99. Diri H, Tanriverdi F, Karaca Z, et al. Extensive investigation of 114 patients with Sheehan's syndrome: a continuing disorder. Eur J Endocrinol 2014;171(3):311–8.

100. Faje A. Hypophysitis: evaluation and management. Clin Diabetes Endocrinol 2016;2:15.
101. Caturegli P, Newschaffer C, Olivi A, et al. Autoimmune hypophysitis. Endocr Rev 2005;26(5):599–614.
102. Kyriacou A, Gnanalingham K, Kearney T. Lymphocytic hypophysitisis: modern day management with limited role for surgery. Pituitary 2017;20(2):241–50.
103. Molitch ME, Gillam MP. Lymphocytic hypophysitis. Horm Res 2007;68(Suppl 5): 145–50.
104. Tirosh A, Hirsch D, Robenshtok E, et al. Variations in clinical and imaging findings by time of diagnosis in females with hypopituitarism attributed to lymphocytic hypophysitis. Endocr Pract 2016;22(4):447–53.
105. Tartaglione T, Chiloiro S, Laino ME, et al. Neuro-radiological features can predict hypopituitarism in primary autoimmune hypophysitis. Pituitary 2018. [Epub ahead of print].
106. Guaraldi F, Giordano R, Grottoli S, et al. Pituitary autoimmunity. Front Horm Res 2017;48:48–68.
107. Chiloiro S, Tartaglione T, Capoluongo ED, et al. Hypophysitis outcome and factors predicting responsiveness to glucocorticoid therapy: a prospective and double-arm study. J Clin Endocrinol Metab 2018;103(10):3877–89.
108. Honegger J, Buchfelder M, Schlaffer S, et al, Pituitary Working Group of the German Society of Endocrinology. Treatment of primary hypophysitis in Germany. J Clin Endocrinol Metab 2015;100(9):3460–9.

Neuro-Ophthalmic Disorders in Pregnancy

Aubrey L. Gilbert, MD, PhD[a], Sashank Prasad, MD[b], Robert M. Mallery, MD[b,c],*

KEYWORDS

- Pregnancy • Neuro-ophthalmology • Postpartum relapse
- Hormonally sensitive tumor

KEY POINTS

- Physiologic changes related to pregnancy may significantly impact neuro-ophthalmic disease.
- Autoimmune disorders generally improve to some degree during pregnancy but can worsen postpartum.
- Hormone-responsive tumors may grow rapidly in pregnancy and cause neuro-ophthalmic symptoms.
- Most diagnostic studies are safe in pregnancy but some should be avoided except in dire circumstances.
- Many neuro-ophthalmic conditions in pregnancy require coordinated care among multiple subspecialists.

The physiologic changes that accompany pregnancy have implications for many different body systems. In pregnancy, blood volume and cardiac output can nearly double, patients gain a large amount of weight over a brief period, extracellular fluid dramatically increases as serum osmolality drops, fibrinolytic activity drops and coagulation factors increase, and cellular immunity diminishes.[1,2] Given that pregnancy is a high-volume, high-flow state with significant weight gain, relative hypercoagulability, and immunosuppression, it follows that neuro-ophthalmic disorders influenced by these factors may be provoked, exacerbated, or in some cases ameliorated by the pregnant state. Several benign alterations occur directly to the eye, including refractive change from hormonally mediated fluid shifts in the cornea, myopic shift and impaired accommodation, and intraocular pressure decrease caused by reduced

The authors have no disclosures regarding commercial or financial conflicts of interest or funding.

[a] Department of Ophthalmology, The Permanente Medical Group, Northern California, 975 Sereno Drive, Vallejo, CA 94589, USA; [b] Department of Neurology, Brigham and Women's Hospital, 60 Fenwood Road, Boston, MA 02115, USA; [c] Department of Ophthalmology, Massachusetts Eye and Ear, 243 Charles Street, Boston, MA 02114, USA
* Corresponding author. Department of Neurology, 60 Fenwood Road, Boston, MA 02115.
E-mail address: rmallery@partners.org

Neurol Clin 37 (2019) 85–102
https://doi.org/10.1016/j.ncl.2018.09.001
0733-8619/19/© 2018 Elsevier Inc. All rights reserved.

episcleral venous pressure and increased aqueous outflow.[3,4] More consequential effects on the visual system may occur from disorders that affect neuro-ophthalmic function, including meningioma, pituitary adenoma, demyelinating disease, myasthenia gravis (MG), thyroid eye disease, idiopathic intracranial hypertension (IIH), cerebral venous sinus thrombosis (CVST), vascular disease, migraine, and cranial neuropathy. This article also details potential neuro-ophthalmic complications of preeclampsia and eclampsia and covers the use of common diagnostic studies during pregnancy.

MENINGIOMA

Meningiomas account for more than one-third of all intracranial tumors and are more common in women than men. They typically present later in life than most pregnancies, but they can present during pregnancy.[5] The incidence of gestational meningioma is estimated to be approximately 5.6 cases out of 100,000 pregnant women.[6] Although meningiomas typically exhibit slow growth, their behavior during pregnancy can be more aggressive.[7] A review of 148 cases of pregnancy-related meningiomas detailed four findings that are more common in pregnancy-related meningiomas compared with those in the general population: (1) parasellar location, (2) anterior circulation blood supply, (3) visual symptoms at presentation, and (4) higher rate of clear cell and chordoid histopathologic features.[8] Increased circulating estrogen, progesterone, and prolactin may mediate rapid growth and vascularization of preexisting tumors.[7,8] Vascular endothelial growth factor may also play a role in tumor expansion.[9] The most growth during pregnancy occurs in the second and third trimesters. Although tumors may shrink after delivery, they may grow again during a subsequent pregnancy.[10,11]

The growth of meningiomas in pregnancy can lead to complicated clinical situations. Size and location determine whether tumor growth is asymptomatic or results in symptoms from direct compression of eloquent neural structures, the development of elevated intracranial pressure, or seizure. The preferred management is usually observation until after delivery,[12] but urgent surgical intervention may be necessary in cases of malignant meningioma, hydrocephalus not amenable to more conventional treatment, or progressively enlarging and potentially life-threatening tumors.[9] Although surgical resection of meningioma during pregnancy may be associated with increased maternal and fetal mortalities, the overall outcomes for the mother and fetus have been found to be similar whether surgery occurs before or after delivery. Coordination of neurosurgery, obstetrics, and neurology/neuro-ophthalmology services is important to ensure optimal management.[7]

PITUITARY DISORDERS

Pituitary anatomy and physiology are altered significantly in pregnancy. The pituitary gland grows steadily, ultimately increasing in volume to twice its baseline before returning to normal by 6 months postpartum.[13] This change is evident on MRI and usually does not cause clinically important deficits, although visual loss can occasionally occur from chiasmal compression in the setting of physiologic enlargement.[14] Other causes of pituitary enlargement during pregnancy include prior adenoma, apoplexy, acute Sheehan syndrome, and lymphocytic hypophysitis (LH).[15] Pituitary height greater than 10 mm and asymmetric enlargement or deviation of the pituitary stalk are features that are atypical for physiologic pituitary enlargement during pregnancy and should raise suspicion of other pathology.[16,17]

Pituitary Adenoma

Previously asymptomatic pituitary adenomas may grow during pregnancy, with a risk of visual loss from optic chiasm compression. All forms of pituitary adenoma may enlarge during pregnancy because of global hyperplasia related to increased serum estrogen levels, but tumor cells of prolactinomas have estrogen receptors, which can result in more substantial increases in size and higher risk for visual loss. The risk of significant tumor growth leading to optic chiasm compression is small (likely <5%) for microadenomas (ie, those measuring <1 cm), and higher for macroadenomas.[18] We recommend visual field testing every trimester in patients with microadenomas, and every 1 to 2 months in patients with macroadenomas in close proximity to or abutting the optic chiasm.[15,18] Serial MRI is not recommended during pregnancy for microadenomas or macroadenomas, and prolactin measurements are not typically recommended for monitoring the growth of prolactinomas.[15]

For treatment of an enlarging prolactinomas, bromocriptine is the preferred dopamine agonist for use during pregnancy, but it crosses the placenta and should be used only if necessary. When used, it is recommended to try to start it after the first trimester.[19] In pregnant patients with visual loss from prolactinoma, bromocriptine has been used without adverse effects on the fetus.[20] For microprolactinomas, dopamine agonists can generally be stopped safely because of the low risk of clinically significant expansion,[21] but the initiation or continuation of bromocriptine may be preferable if the tumor is large, particularly if it extends outside the sella.[18] Although dopamine agonists are also safe for the breastfeeding infant, these medications impair lactation. Unless required to prevent tumor growth, dopamine agonists should be avoided in women who wish to breastfeed.[22]

Surgical intervention, generally via a transsphenoidal approach in the second trimester, is usually not required unless there are significant deficits from compression of the optic chiasm. Most women with prolactinomas and nonfunctioning adenomas have good pregnancy outcomes, but rarely, apoplexy occurs.[20,23] As in cases of meningioma during pregnancy, management of adenoma should be guided by a collaborative approach involving multiple subspecialists, particularly including an endocrinologist.

Lymphocytic Hypophysitis

LH may also result in pituitary enlargement during pregnancy. Approximately 50% to 60% of all women with LH present during pregnancy or postpartum, usually in the last month of gestation or within 2 months postpartum.[24] Patients typically present with symptoms of hypopituitarism and mass effect (headache, visual loss). Diabetes insipidus and mild elevation in prolactin may be present, and the latter may interfere with lactation.[25,26] The underlying pathology is a lymphocytic infiltration of the gland with varying degrees of dysfunction based on the structures affected; anterior, posterior, or pan-hypophysitis can occur.[27] The mechanism of this disorder is unknown, but it is thought to be driven by abnormal autoimmunity. Theories regarding the link to pregnancy include the release of pituitary antigens, increased immune system access to the gland, and placental cross-reactivity.[15]

LH may be mistaken for pituitary adenoma or Sheehan syndrome in some cases (**Fig. 1**). Imaging of LH often reveals diffuse thickening of the pituitary stalk. When performed with contrast, MRI shows higher than normal contrast enhancement of the gland and loss of the neurohypophyseal bright spot on unenhanced T1-weighted images.[28,29] Additional clues for separating LH from adenoma are symmetric pituitary enlargement, a thickened but nondeviated stalk, a uniformly flat sellar floor, and the appearance of a dural tail (representing contrast enhancement of adjacent dura).[30]

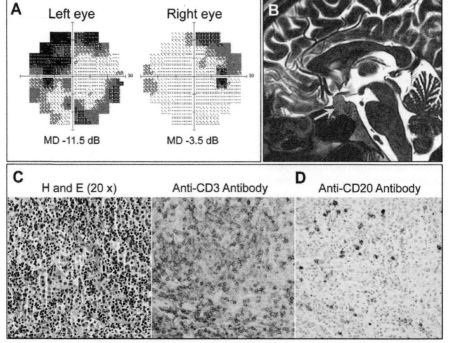

Fig. 1. A 32-year-old pregnant (29 weeks, 5 days) woman who presented with headache and visual loss related to lymphocytic hypophysitis. (*A*) Automated visual field testing showed bilateral visual field loss greatest in the superior temporal quadrant of the right eye and the superior-temporal quadrant of the left eye. (*B*) Sagittal T2-weighted MRI showed enlargement of the pituitary gland (*yellow arrow*; 1.2 cm in craniocaudal dimension) with superior displacement of the optic chiasm (*red arrowhead*). Gadolinium contrast was not given because of the pregnancy. (*C*) The patient underwent endoscopic transnasal-transsphenoidal partial resection of the lesion, with pathology demonstrating anterior pituitary tissue densely infiltrated by lymphoplasmocytic cells. CD3 immunostain showed these were predominantly small CD3-immunoreactive T lymphocytes. (*D*) CD20-positive B lymphocytes were uncommon, excluding lymphoma. The patient's vision recovered fully, and 1 year after presentation, the patient remains with secondary adrenal insufficiency and central hypothyroidism. (*Courtesy of* Dr Jasmin Lebastchi, Boston, MA; with permission.)

Replacement of hormonal deficiencies is the mainstay of treatment of LH,[15] but pharmacologic dosing of corticosteroids may lead to improved anterior pituitary insufficiency in comparison with replacement of physiologic cortisol doses.[31] Surgical intervention is reserved for cases of visual or neurologic impairment.

DEMYELINATING DISEASE

The physiologic immunosuppression of pregnancy is intended to prevent the mother's immune system from targeting the fetus. Because the changes that occur primarily affect cellular immune function, diseases that are immune-mediated may improve during pregnancy.[32,33] After delivery, however, autoimmune disorders may worsen, and women who have had improvement during pregnancy may experience clinical relapses postpartum.[34–36]

Multiple Sclerosis

Multiple sclerosis (MS) is an inflammatory demyelinating disease of the central nervous system that occurs most commonly in women of childbearing age. Pregnancy is not typically considered to be high risk in these patients because it does not alter the overall disease course or disability progression.[37,38] Although MS generally improves during pregnancy, with a decreased relapse rate particularly in the third trimester, there is an increased risk of relapse postpartum. It is thus important to stabilize disease activity before patients attempt to become pregnant.[39] MS has no clear negative effects on pregnancy or fetal outcomes, but all disease-modifying therapies have some potential downside for fertility or pregnancy outcomes. Evidence suggests that interferon-β (Food and Drug Administration [FDA] class C, unknown risk) and glatiramer acetate (FDA class B, no evidence of risk apparent in humans) are safe to use throughout pregnancy, with little effect on the fetus. However, immunosuppressive drugs are often held during pregnancy and for some time before conception, and then resumed immediately postpartum to mitigate relapse. Avoidance of breastfeeding while on disease-modifying therapies is recommended.[37,39]

Neuromyelitis Optica

Neuromyelitis optica (NMO) is another inflammatory demyelinating central nervous system disease that often affects women of childbearing age. Aquaporin-4 (AQP4)-IgG, an autoantibody against an astrocytic water channel protein, is believed to play a key role in the pathogenesis of NMO via complement-mediated astrocyte damage with inflammatory infiltrate and loss of myelin.[40] Patients typically present with severe optic neuritis, transverse myelitis, or both. Although AQP4-IgG has been found to transfer from mother to fetus, this does not seem to cause disease in the child.[41]

Although there may be some decrease in NMO activity during pregnancy, this occurs to a much lesser degree than in MS.[36] Like MS, however, there is a marked increase in relapse rate immediately postpartum (**Fig. 2**), particularly in the initial 3 to 6 months after delivery; patients with high levels of disease activity before pregnancy are more likely to have pregnancy-related relapses.[42,43] The elevated estrogen levels associated with pregnancy can increase disease activity by decreasing apoptosis of self-reactive B cells, facilitating development of new self-reactive peripheral B cells, and shifting the balance toward TH2-mediated immunity.[42]

In addition to postpartum disease activity, patients with NMO have increased rates of miscarriage and preeclampsia. Placental trophoblasts express AQP4 antigen, and animal models have shown that the placenta is a site of maternal AQP4-IgG antibody binding, complement deposition, and placental necrosis.[40] Nour and colleagues[44] reviewed the cases of 60 AQP4-IgG-positive NMO spectrum disorder patients who became pregnant and found an increased rate of miscarriage after NMO spectrum disorder onset (43%) compared with before (7%). They noted that higher disease activity seemed to precede pregnancies that ended in miscarriage. Although they also found that the risk of preeclampsia was higher in these women than in the general population (11% vs 3%), this did not increase after NMO spectrum disorder onset.

Chronic immunosuppression is the foundation for management of NMO, and cessation or decreasing of immunosuppressive regimens seems to be partly responsible for the increased risk of relapse postpartum.[45] Depending on the agent, it may be favorable to continue immunosuppression through pregnancy,[41] but certain medications should be discontinued before conception (mycophenolate mofetil 6 weeks prior, and methotrexate and cyclophosphamide 3 months prior). Several alternative treatment options are safe during pregnancy, particularly azathioprine and rituximab,

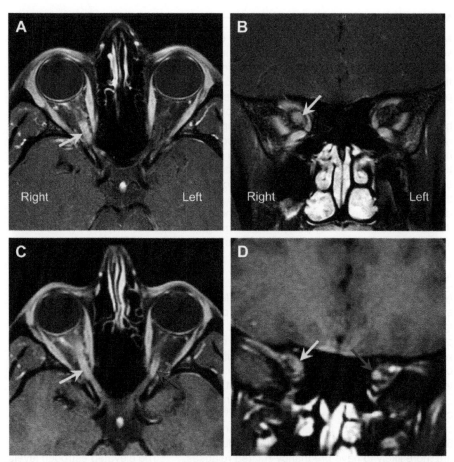

Fig. 2. A 30-year-old woman who presented with sequential optic neuritis at 1 month post-partum. (*A, B*) Initially, the patient's visual acuities measured counting fingers in the right eye and 20/20 in the left eye. T1-weighted postcontrast axial and coronal images showed enhancement of the right intraorbital optic nerve (*yellow arrows*). (*C, D*) Twelve days later she developed visual loss in the left eye, with visual acuities measuring light perception in the right eye and hand motion in the left eye. Repeat MRI showed new enhancement of the left optic nerve (*red arrows*) in addition to more extensive enhancement of the right optic nerve (*yellow arrows*). Serum testing for aquaporin-4 immunoglobulin G was positive, confirming the diagnosis of neuromyelitis optica.

and these decrease the risk of relapse through pregnancy and after delivery. Myco-phenolate mofetil, methotrexate, and cyclophosphamide should also be avoided during breastfeeding, and it is recommended to wait 4 hours to breastfeed after taking azathioprine. It may be preferable for patients at high risk of relapse to forgo breast-feeding in favor of optimal immunosuppression.[41]

For acute exacerbations during pregnancy, corticosteroids and plasma exchange may be used safely. Corticosteroids should be used at the lowest possible effective doses, and patients should be monitored for gestational diabetes if they require prolonged corticosteroid use. Stress dose steroids should also be provided before delivery to patients who have been on steroid treatment for more than 2 weeks.[41]

MYASTHENIA GRAVIS

MG is another autoimmune disorder that is common in young women of childbearing age. It affects almost 1 million people worldwide, is typically diagnosed in the second or third decade of life, and is twice as common in women as in men.[46,47] Its underlying pathology is dysfunction of neuromuscular transmission caused by antibodies targeting components of the neuromuscular junction, most commonly the acetylcholine receptor. The most common neuro-ophthalmic symptoms are fatigable ptosis and diplopia with variable abnormalities in extraocular movements, but the disease may be life-threatening in cases of respiratory muscle compromise. The course of MG in pregnancy is unpredictable, and it may vary from one pregnancy to the next. The highest periods of risk for disease exacerbation are usually the first trimester and the first month postpartum, whereas 20% to 40% of women experience improvement in their second and third trimesters.[48–50] In myasthenic women who are pregnant or recently pregnant, there is an inverse correlation between mortality risk and disease duration, with the highest mortality risk in the first year after disease onset and the lowest risk after 7 years.[50]

Treatment of MG during pregnancy must be tailored to the individual patient. Some patients with mild disease may go through pregnancy without treatment. Doses of up to 600 mg/d of pyridostigmine are considered safe in pregnancy. Because of changes in absorption, dosages may require frequent adjustment. Pyridostigmine can be administered intravenously in cases of hyperemesis gravidarum, but in this form it can cause uterine contractions and premature labor. Steroids may be used when needed. The dosage should be minimized, and patients should be monitored carefully for gestational diabetes.[50,51] The use of immunosuppressive medications is difficult in pregnancy, but guidelines permit using azathioprine throughout pregnancy and breastfeeding. Although azathioprine crosses the placenta, the fetus is unable to convert it to active metabolites and is therefore largely protected from its effects[52]; however, some neonatal side effects have been reported, including thrombocytopenia, anemia, leukopenia, thymic atrophy, decreased immunoglobulin levels, and increased risk of immunosuppression. Cyclosporin A can also be used during pregnancy and breastfeeding but carries risks of prematurity, low birth weight, and spontaneous abortion.[50,52] Mycophenolate mofetil should be discontinued at least 6 weeks before conception. Although thymectomy during pregnancy is not routinely recommended, acute exacerbations are safely treated with plasma exchange and immunoglobulin therapy.[50]

There are some additional considerations pertaining to the peripartum period and delivery in myasthenic patients. Assistance may be required for supranormal fatigue during delivery, but this is usually in the form of forceps or vacuum. Cesarean section is still reserved for general obstetric considerations.[50,53] Nevertheless, women with MG may have greater rates of preterm premature rupture of membranes and cesarean delivery.[54] Myasthenic patients can also have heightened sensitivity to certain anesthetics, and ester-type medications should be avoided because they can exacerbate the disease.[55] Similarly, magnesium is contraindicated for eclampsia management in MG patients because it inhibits acetylcholine release and may cause acute worsening.[56]

Neonatal Myasthenia Gravis

A total of 10% to 20% of neonates born to myasthenic mothers have transient myasthenic symptoms, such as ptosis, a weak cry, facial weakness, poor sucking, hypotonia, and respiratory distress, usually occurring within the first few days of life and resolving within a month, because of transplacental conveyance of maternal anti-bodies.[57] This is less common in seronegative mothers,[57–59] but can still occur and may occur later in this setting.[60] Neonates with significant respiratory compromise may require mechanical ventilation, pyridostigmine, and/or plasma exchange.[56,61] Breastfeeding is not contraindicated for mothers with MG unless they are on certain immunosuppressive medications. Because the acetylcholine receptor antibodies are secreted in breastmilk, it carries the risk of transient neonatal myasthenia, and infants and mothers should be monitored closely for symptoms postpartum.[50] Pyrido-stigmine, steroids, and azathioprine are considered safe during lactation, although high doses of pyridostigmine may cause stomach upset in the infant.[50] Mycopheno-late mofetil should not be used while breastfeeding.[50,55]

THYROID ORBITOPATHY

Patients with thyroid orbitopathy may experience diplopia or visual impairment from compressive optic neuropathy secondary to inflammatory intraorbital changes and enlargement of the extraocular muscles. Thyroid orbitopathy is most commonly associated with Graves hyperthyroidism, which generally improves to some degree during gestation and rebounds postpartum. It is thus not surprising that antithyroid antibody titers have been found to decrease during pregnancy and to rise postpartum, although these do not always correlate to the severity of the orbital reaction.[62] It has also been speculated that changes in the function of the thyroid-stimulating hormone receptor (from stimulating to blocking) may occur during pregnancy.[63]

Maintaining a euthyroid state is optimal in pregnant patients with thyroid orbitop-athy, and although antithyroid medications cross the placenta and do affect fetal hor-mone production, pharmacologic therapy is still the treatment of choice for hyperthyroidism during pregnancy. Thyroid function must be monitored closely because dysfunction can lead to significant fetal morbidity.[63] Although rare, severe orbitopathy can occur in pregnancy even under euthyroid conditions, requiring more aggressive management with steroids or surgical intervention.[64]

IDIOPATHIC INTRACRANIAL HYPERTENSION

IIH is a disease characterized by elevated intracranial pressure in the absence of infec-tion, inflammation, thrombosis, or mass. Typically, patients are obese women of child-bearing age, and present with headache, pulsatile tinnitus, and blurred vision related to papilledema (**Fig. 3**). Occasionally patients develop diplopia secondary to sixth cra-nial nerve palsy. Depending on the degree of papilledema and whether there is a fulmi-nant course, vision loss may range from none to severe. IIH is not more frequent in pregnancy, but women with previously diagnosed IIH may experience worsening dur-ing pregnancy because of weight gain.[65]

Acetazolamide and topiramate are the primary medical therapies for IIH. In general, the use of these medications is avoided during pregnancy, but acetazolamide (FDA class C) can be used in cases with vision-threatening disease.[66–68] Although at high doses in animal studies acetazolamide may produce birth defects (forelimb anomalies in rats, mice, and hamsters) there is little evidence to support any adverse effect in hu-man pregnancy.[68] In a retrospective, case-control study including 101 women with IIH and a total of 158 pregnancies, of which 50 involved acetazolamide usage before 13 weeks of gestation, for acetazolamide users the risk of spontaneous abortion was similar to the control group, and no major complication was identified in their in-fants.[67] It has thus been suggested that acetazolamide may be used in pregnancy in appropriate clinical situations as long as patients are properly informed of potential

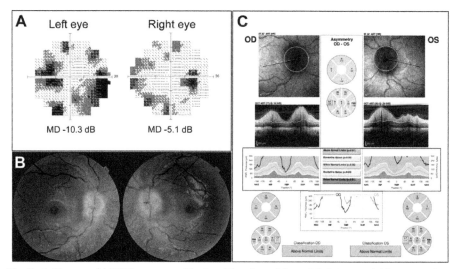

Fig. 3. A 22-year-old G1P0 woman with visual loss from idiopathic intracranial hypertension. She developed headaches at 10 weeks of pregnancy and was found to have papilledema. MRI brain, MRV (Magnetic Resonance Venogram) head, and lumbar puncture (opening pressure 33 cm H_2O and normal constituents) confirmed the diagnosis, and acetazolamide, 250 mg BID, was started at 15 weeks. She presented to neuro-ophthalmology clinic at 30 weeks. (*A*) Automated perimetry showed bilateral blind spot enlargement and nasal depressions, worse in the left eye. (*B*) Fundus examination showed chronic-appearing grade 3 papilledema OD and grade 3 papilledema OS. (*C*) Optical coherence tomography allows the precise measurement of retinal nerve fiber layer edema. The peripapillary retinal nerve fiber layer thickness is plotted (within the *red box*) in comparison with the normal reference range (*green region*) in each eye. There was marked thickening of the peripapillary retinal nerve fiber layer bilaterally. With an increase in the patient's acetazolamide dose to 1000 mg twice daily and weight loss, the patient's visual fields and papilledema improved during the remainder of her pregnancy.

risks.[68] Topiramate is FDA class D and should not be used in pregnancy because it is associated with cleft lip and cleft palate when taken in the first trimester.[69] Furosemide, which is occasionally used in acetazolamide-intolerant patients or as a supplement to acetazolamide, is also FDA class C.

In refractory cases close to delivery, some practitioners recommend serial lumbar punctures as a temporizing measure, although the ameliorative effects are often short-lived.[3] In cases of progressive visual loss, refractory to medical treatment, optic nerve sheath fenestration or cerebrospinal fluid diversion procedures (lumbar-peritoneal or ventriculoperitoneal shunting) may be necessary.[70] Ultimately, the risk of visual loss is the same in pregnant and nonpregnant women with IIH,[71] and subsequent pregnancies do not increase the risk of recurrence.[70] Although intracranial pressure can increase up to 70 cm H_2O with Valsalva during labor,[72,73] IIH is generally not an indication for cesarean section and delivery mode is instead determined by obstetric factors.[71]

CEREBRAL VENOUS SINUS THROMBOSIS

Because pregnancy is a hypercoagulable state, pregnant women are at increased risk for occlusive vascular disorders. In pregnant women, the incidence of CVST is estimated between 100 and 1000 per million per year, whereas the incidence of CVST in the general population is between 13 and 19 per million per year.[3,74,75] CVST can present similarly to IIH, with headache and papilledema. Patients can also have seizures and more significant neurologic sequelae, including venous stroke or hemorrhage.[76] Hyperemesis gravidarum, hypertension, advanced maternal age, delivery by cesarean section, and infection all increase the risk of venous sinus thrombosis in pregnant women. Underlying hypercoagulable disorders, including inherited thrombophilia, or acquired conditions, such as antiphospholipid syndrome, are also important considerations.

The diagnosis of CVST is confirmed using magnetic resonance or computed tomographic angiography. Whether pregnant or not, patients with CVST should be treated with anticoagulation, usually initially with intravenous unfractionated heparin, but thrombolysis or thrombectomy is considered in those cases with neurologic deterioration.[77,78] Heparin significantly decreases the risk of death in pregnant women with CVST, without significant maternal or fetal side effects.[79,80] Acetazolamide may also be used to lower intracranial pressure in patients with significant visual loss related to papilledema.

After the acute treatment, the patient is transitioned to a low-molecular-weight heparin (eg, enoxaparin, FDA class B) given in therapeutic doses subcutaneously. Warfarin should not be used in pregnancy because it is FDA class X, but it can be used during lactation postpartum. Fortunately, it has been shown that recurrent venous thrombotic events during subsequent pregnancies are infrequent.[81] It is recommended that estrogen-containing contraceptives be avoided in women who have suffered a previous CVST. Although subsequent pregnancies are considered safe, consideration should be given to the use of low-molecular-weight heparin prophylactically during gestation and peripartum.[77]

STROKE

Pregnant women have an increased risk of stroke because of altered hemodynamics and coagulability, and cerebrovascular disease accounts for up to 6% of maternal mortality.[82] Cerebral infarction may have neuro-ophthalmic consequences by affecting parts of the visual or ocular motor pathways, including the retina. In a retrospective review of more than 7 million deliveries in the United States during 1993 and 1994, Kittner and colleagues[83] reported 13.1 cases of stroke per 100,000 deliveries. Factors associated with the stroke occurrence included hypertension, fluid and electrolyte imbalance, acid-base disorders, and cesarean delivery. Rarely, amniotic fluid embolism can occur peripartum and occlude multiple arterioles.[84] Both evaluation for the cause of stroke and acute therapy should proceed as it would for a nonpregnant patient.[85]

Hemorrhagic strokes can also occur during pregnancy in the setting of ruptured aneurysm or arteriovenous malformation. There is considerable debate, however, as to whether the risk of rupture is elevated in pregnancy, with some arguing that it is[86–88] and others arguing that it is not.[89–91]

MIGRAINE

The lifetime prevalence of migraine in women is reported to range between 16% and 32%, rising after the average age of menarche, and peaking before the average age of menopause. Thus, migraine commonly affects women during childbearing years.[92] Migraine patients may present to neuro-ophthalmologists if their migraines are associated with visual aura. Although most women with migraine (60%–87%) see improvement during pregnancy (especially in the second and third trimester),[93] a small percentage (4%–8%) may worsen, particularly those with a history of migraine aura.[94] Some women may also experience migraine for the first time during pregnancy (usually in the first trimester), and many of these women have aura.[95] Migraine symptoms also often increase postpartum as estrogen decreases rapidly, but breastfeeding may delay their return by keeping estrogen levels higher.[94]

Most preventative medications for chronic migraine are FDA class C or worse, and the decision to use these agents should involve discussion with the patient and their obstetrician. Propranolol, verapamil, and gabapentin are FDA class C, and there are data suggesting fetal risk with the use of topiramate (FDA class D), valproic acid (FDA class D for epilepsy; FDA class X when used for migraine), tricyclic antidepressants (FDA class C), and candesartan (FDA class D for hypertension; FDA class X when used for migraine).[94] Lifestyle changes or nonmedical treatments, such as acupuncture, heat or ice packs, meditation, and exercise, are the first line of treatment in many cases.[96] Riboflavin (vitamin B_2) may help reduce migraine frequency and has no known toxicities, and magnesium is FDA class A.

For acute migraine therapy, limited use of caffeine and acetaminophen (FDA class B) may be considered. Nonsteroidal anti-inflammatory drugs are used sparingly in early pregnancy, but become FDA class D can be in the third trimester. There are a handful of FDA class B antiemetic drugs that may be used for migraine-associated nausea, but ginger may also be an alternative.[97] For severe migraine attacks, intravenous hydration and antiemetics are helpful, and as well as intranasal lidocaine (FDA class B). Triptans (serotonin 1b/1d agonists) are FDA class C.

It is important to keep in mind that pregnant women with migraine may have increased risk of hypertension, preeclampsia, fetal growth restriction, placental abruption, and arterial and venous thrombosis.[98–100]

CRANIAL NEUROPATHY

Cranial neuropathies can occur in the setting of many of the disease processes detailed in this review. Isolated idiopathic cranial neuropathies also occur during pregnancy. The most common of these is facial nerve palsy, followed by abducens and then trochlear nerve palsy.[3] Idiopathic trigeminal or oculomotor palsy occurs rarely. Facial nerve palsies in pregnancy have classically been attributed to increased pressure on the nerve from interstitial fluid.[101] Most cases of facial palsy occur in the second and third trimesters,[102] with outcomes reportedly worse for those cases that arise late in pregnancy or early in the postpartum period.[103] Recent recommendations suggest assessment for atypical causes, and early introduction of corticosteroids to limit progression and improve prognosis in these cases.[102] Abducens palsy may be idiopathic in pregnancy but more commonly has been associated with gestational hypertension or preeclampsia.[104,105] Some of the trochlear nerve palsies reported in pregnancy may represent decompensations of congenital palsies.[106] Transient trigeminal palsy and Horner syndrome have also been reported after epidural analgesia, and Horner syndrome may be more common after epidural block in pregnant women than in nonpregnant women.[107] A recent review of cranial nerve palsies following neuraxial block in pregnancy identified only abducens and facial palsies. Around 58% (25/43 cases) followed epidural block, around 26% (11/43 cases) were after spinal anesthesia, and around 16% (7/43 cases) were after combined spinal-epidural anesthesia. Post-dural puncture headache preceded the palsy in most cases, and intracranial hypotension was believed to be the most common cause for the palsies. Some of the cases were treated with epidural blood patches, and most (81%) patients had complete resolution within weeks to months. It is still recommended to obtain neuroimaging in every case to avoid missing other etiologies.[108] A rare presentation of isolated oculomotor nerve palsy has been reported in pregnancy in association with eclampsia.[109] A case of multiple cranial neuropathies in the setting of preeclampsia has also been reported.[110]

PREECLAMPSIA AND ECLAMPSIA

Preeclampsia and eclampsia are pregnancy-specific states that can occur in the second half of gestation. Preeclampsia is diagnosed by the presence of hypertension and proteinuria; eclampsia may follow and is defined by the presence of seizure and/or coma. About one-quarter of patients with severe preeclampsia have visual changes that can include diplopia, scotoma, or photopsia.[3,11] In addition to multiple retinal findings including hypertensive retinopathy, serous retinal detachment, and choroidal infarction, patients with severe manifestations of pre/eclampsia may develop optic disc edema. Patients often experience retinal vasospasm,[112] and nonarteritic ischemic optic neuropathy has also been reported.[113,114] Cortical visual loss may result from posterior reversible encephalopathy syndrome or stroke.[115–117] Definitive treatment of severe preeclampsia and eclampsia is delivery of the baby, but intravenous magnesium sulfate may also be used as an anticonvulsant, to counteract cerebral vasospasm, and to tighten the cerebral blood-brain barrier and reduce cerebral edema.[118,119] Potential neuro-ophthalmic side effects of magnesium sulfate include impaired accommodation, impaired convergence, and ptosis.[111]

USE OF COMMON DIAGNOSTIC STUDIES AND EYE DROPS DURING PREGNANCY

Assuming none of the normal contraindications, MRI is considered safe and the imaging modality of choice in pregnancy, but all FDA-approved gadolinium chelates are FDA class C. Gadolinium is thus reserved for cases absolutely requiring it to evaluate potentially life-threatening outcomes for the fetus or the mother and, even then, it is typically avoided until after the first trimester.[120,121] Breastfeeding after gadolinium, however, is acceptable.[121] Computed tomography scans are done with appropriate abdominal shielding, but radiation exposure should be minimized, particularly early in pregnancy. Iodinated contrast dye is class B (animal studies show risk but no definite evidence of risk is apparent in humans). Catheter angiography can be done in pregnancy without elevated risk.[122] Lumbar puncture is safe in pregnancy barring any of the normal contraindications. Although fluorescein and indocyanine green used in retinal angiography are class C, fluorescein crosses the placenta and also enters breast milk, whereas indocyanine green does neither.[3,123–125] Although no teratogenic effects have been reported from the use of dilating drops or topical anesthetic during pregnancy, systemic use of atropine, homatropine, or phenylephrine should be avoided in early pregnancy because these have been associated with fetal malformations.[66]

SUMMARY

Physiologic changes related to pregnancy may significantly impact neuro-ophthalmic disease, and special consideration must be given to evaluation and management of pregnant patients presenting with visual complaints and to patients with preexisting neuro-ophthalmic disease who are contemplating pregnancy. Knowledge of potential complications affecting patients with neuro-ophthalmic disease in pregnancy and the safety profiles of various medications and studies can help optimize counseling and care.

REFERENCES

1. Carlin A, Alfirevic Z. Physiological changes of pregnancy and monitoring. Best Pract Res Clin Obstet Gynaecol 2008;22:801–23.
2. Thornburg KL, Jacobson SL, Giraud GD, et al. Hemodynamic changes in pregnancy. Semin Perinatol 2000;24:11–4.
3. Digre, Kathleen B. Neuro-ophthalmology and pregnancy: what does a neuro-ophthalmologist need to know? J Neuroophthalmol 2011;31(4):381–7.
4. Sharma S, Wuntakal R, Anand A, et al. Pregnancy and the eye. Obstet Gynaecol 2006;8:141–6.
5. Wiemels J, Wrensch M, Claus EB. Epidemiology and etiology of meningioma. J Neurooncol 2010;99(3):307–14.
6. Dumitrescu BC, Tataranu LG, Gorgan MR. Pregnant woman with an intracranial meningioma: case report and review of the literature. Rom J Neurosurg 2014;21: 489–96.
7. Wan WL, Geller JL, Feldon SE, et al. Visual loss caused by rapidly progressive intracranial meningiomas during pregnancy. Ophthalmology 1990;97:18–21.
8. Laviv Y, Ohla V, Kasper ME. Unique features of pregnancy-related meningiomas: lessons learned from 148 reported cases and theoretical implications of a prolactin modulated pathogenesis. Neurosurg Rev 2018;41(1):95–108.
9. Hortobagyi T, Bencze J, Murnyak B, et al. Pathophysiology of meningioma growth in pregnancy. Open Med (Wars) 2017;12:195–200.
10. Cushing H, Eisenhardt L. Meningiomas arising from the tuberculum sellae. Arch Ophthalmol 1929;1:168–205.
11. Chow MS, Mercier PA, Omahen DA, et al. Recurrent exophytic meningioma in pregnancy. Obstet Gynecol 2013;121(2 Pt 2 Suppl 1):475–8.
12. Finfer SR. Management of labour and delivery in patients with intracranial neoplasms. Br J Anaesth 1991;67:784–7.
13. Dinç H, Esen F, Demirci A, et al. Pituitary dimensions and volume measurements in pregnancy and post partum. MR assessment. Acta Radiol 1998;39(1):64–9.
14. Inoue T, Hotta A, Awai M, et al. Loss of vision due to a physiologic pituitary enlargement during normal pregnancy. Graefes Arch Clin Exp Ophthalmol 2007;245:1049–51.
15. Karaca Z, Tanriverdi F, Unluhizarci K, et al. Pregnancy and pituitary disorders. Eur J Endocrinol 2010;162:453–75.
16. Wolpert SM, Molitch ME, Goldman JA, et al. Size, shape, and appearance of the normal female pituitary gland. Am J Roentgenol 1984;143:377–81.
17. Elster AD, Sanders TG, Vines FS, et al. Size and shape of the pituitary gland during pregnancy and postpartum: measurement with MR imaging. Radiology 1991;181:531–5.
18. Kupersmith MJ, Rosenberg C, Kleinberg D. Visual loss in pregnant women with pituitary adenomas. Ann Intern Med 1994;121:473–7.
19. Sam S, Molitch ME. Timing and special concerns regarding endocrine surgery during pregnancy. Endocrinol Metab Clin North Am 2003;32:337–54.
20. Galvão A, Gonçalves D, Moreira M, et al. Prolactinoma and pregnancy: a series of cases including pituitary apoplexy. J Obstet Gynaecol 2017;37(3):284–7.
21. Musolino NRC, Bronstein MD. Prolactinomas and pregnancy. In: Bronstein MD, editor. Pituitary tumors in pregnancy. Boston: Kluwer Academic Publishers; 2001. p. 91–108.

22. Bronstein MD, Salgado LR, Castro Musolino NR. Medical management of pituitary adenomas: the special case of management of the pregnant woman. Pituitary 2002;5:99–107.
23. Lambert K, Rees K, Seed PT, et al. Macroprolactinomas and nonfunctioning pituitary adenomas and pregnancy outcomes. Obstet Gynecol 2017;129(1): 185–94.
24. Beressi N, Beressi JP, Cohen R, et al. Lymphocytic hypophysitis. A review of 145 cases. Ann Med Interne 1999;150:327–41.
25. Molitch ME. Pituitary disorders during pregnancy. Endocrinol Metab Clin North Am 2006;35:99–116.
26. Patel MC, Guneratne N, Haq N, et al. Peripartum hypopituitarism and lymphocytic hypophysitis. Q J Med 1995;88:571–80.
27. Rivera JA. Lymphocytic hypophysitis: disease spectrum and approach to diagnosis and therapy. Pituitary 2006;9:35–45.
28. Imura H, Nakao K, Shimatsu A, et al. Lymphocytic infundibuloneurohypophysitis as a cause of central diabetes insipidus. N Engl J Med 1993;329:683–9.
29. Leggett DA, Hill PT, Anderson RJ. 'Stalkitis' in a pregnant 32-year-old woman: a rare cause of diabetes insipidus. Australas Radiol 1999;43:104–17.
30. Bellastella A, Bizzarro A, Coronella C, et al. Lymphocytic hypophysitis: a rare or underestimated disease? Eur J Endocrinol 2003;149:363–76.
31. Wang S, Wang L, Yao Y, et al. Primary lymphocytic hypophysitis: clinical characteristics and treatment of 50 cases in a single centre in China over 18 years. Clin Endocrinol (Oxf) 2017;87(2):177–84.
32. Martin C, Varner MW. Physiologic changes in pregnancy: surgical implications. Clin Obstet Gynecol 1994;37:241–55.
33. Aagaard-Tillery KM, Silver R, Dalton J. Immunology of normal pregnancy. Semin Fetal Neonatal Med 2006;11:279–95.
34. Neuteboom RF, Janssens AC, Siepman TA, et al. Pregnancy in multiple sclerosis: clinical and self-report scales. J Neurol 2012;259(2):311–7.
35. Vukusic S, Hutchinson M, Hours M, et al. Pregnancy and multiple sclerosis (the PRIMS study): clinical predictors of post-partum relapse. Brain 2004;127: 1353–60.
36. Klawiter EC, Bove R, Elsone L, et al. High risk of postpartum relapses in neuromyelitis optica spectrum disorder. Neurology 2017;89(22):2238–44.
37. Pozzilli C, Pugliatti M, ParadigMS Group. An overview of pregnancy-related issues in patients with multiple sclerosis. Eur J Neurol 2015;22(Suppl 2):34–9.
38. Confavreux C, Hutchinson M, Hours MM, et al. Rate of pregnancy-related relapse in multiple sclerosis. Pregnancy in Multiple Sclerosis Group. N Engl J Med 1998;339(5):285–91.
39. Shimizu Y. Management of multiple sclerosis and neuromyelitis optica in pregnancy and childbearing. Clin Exp Neuroimmunol 2015;6:93–8.
40. Saadoun S, Waters P, Leite MI, et al. Neuromyelitis optica IgG causes placental inflammation and fetal death. J Immunol 2013;191(6):2999–3005.
41. Shosha E, Pittock SJ, Flanagan E, et al. Neuromyelitis optica spectrum disorders and pregnancy: interactions and management. Mult Scler 2017;23(14): 1808–17.
42. Davoudi V, Keyhanian K, Bove RM, et al. Immunology of neuromyelitis optica during pregnancy. Neurol Neuroimmunol Neuroinflamm 2016;3(6):e288.
43. Kim W, Kim SH, Nakashima I, et al. Influence of pregnancy on neuromyelitis optica spectrum disorder. Neurology 2012;78(16):1264–7.

44. Nour MM, Nakashima I, Coutinho E, et al. Pregnancy outcomes in aquaporin-4-positive neuromyelitis optica spectrum disorder. Neurology 2016;86(1):79–87.
45. Shimizu Y, Fujihara K, Ohashi T, et al. Pregnancy-related relapse risk factors in women with anti-AQP4 antibody positivity and neuromyelitis optica spectrum disorder. Mult Scler 2016;22(11):1413–20.
46. Gilhus NE, Owe JF, Hoff JM, et al. Myasthenia gravis: a review of available treatment approaches. Autoimmune Dis 2011;2011:847393.
47. Ferrero S, Esposito F, Biamonti M, et al. Myasthenia gravis during pregnancy. Expert Rev Neurother 2008;8(6):979–88.
48. Batocchi AP, Majolini L, Evoli A, et al. Course and treatment of myasthenia gravis during pregnancy. Neurology 1999;52:447–52.
49. Djelmis J, Sostarko M, Mayer D, et al. Myasthenia gravis in pregnancy: report on 69 cases. Eur J Obstet Gynecol Reprod Biol 2002;104:21–5.
50. Ferrero S, Pretta S, Nicoletti A, et al. Myasthenia gravis: management issues during pregnancy. Eur J Obstet Gynecol Reprod Biol 2005;121:129–38.
51. Hoff JM, Daltveit AK, Gilhus NE. Myasthenia gravis in pregnancy and birth: identifying risk factors, optimising care. Eur J Neurol 2007;14:38–43.
52. Norwood F, Dhanjal M, Hill M, et al. Myasthenia in pregnancy: best practice guidelines from a U.K. multispecialty working group. J Neurol Neurosurg Psychiatry 2014;85:538–43.
53. Hassan A, Yasawy ZM. Myasthaenia gravis: clinical management issues before, during and after pregnancy. Sultan Qaboos Univ Med J 2017;17(3):e259–67.
54. Ducci RD, Lorenzoni PJ, Kay CSK, et al. Clinical follow-up of pregnancy in myasthenia gravis patients. Neuromuscul Disord 2017;(27):352–7.
55. Varner M. Myasthenia gravis and pregnancy. Clin Obstet Gynecol 2013;56:372–81.
56. Massey JM, De Jesus-Acosta C. Pregnancy and myasthenia gravis. Continuum (Minneap Minn) 2014;20:115–27.
57. Ciafaloni E, Massey JM. Myasthenia gravis and pregnancy. Neurol Clin 2004;22:771–82.
58. O'Carroll P, Bertorini TE, Jacob G, et al. Transient neonatal myasthenia in a baby born to a mother with new-onset anti-MuSK-mediated myasthenia gravis. J Clin Neuromuscul Dis 2009;11:69–71.
59. Niks EH, Verrips A, Semmekrot BA, et al. A transient neonatal myasthenic syndrome with anti-musk antibodies. Neurology 2008;70:1215–6.
60. Townsel C, Keller R, Johnson K, et al. Seronegative maternal ocular myasthenia gravis and delayed transient neonatal myasthenia gravis. AJP Rep 2016;6:e133–6.
61. Hamel J, Ciafaloni E. An update: myasthenia gravis and pregnancy. Neurol Clin 2018;36(2):355–65.
62. Wall JR, Lahooti H, Hibbert EJ, et al. Relationship between clinical and immunological features of thyroid autoimmunity and ophthalmopathy during pregnancy. J Thyroid Res 2015;2015:698470.
63. Bucci I, Giuliani C, Napolitano G. Thyroid-stimulating hormone receptor antibodies in pregnancy: clinical relevance. Front Endocrinol (Lausanne) 2017;8:137.
64. Stafford IP, Dildy GA 3rd, Miller JM Jr. Severe Graves' ophthalmopathy in pregnancy. Obstet Gynecol 2005;105(5 Pt 2):1221–3.
65. Kassam SH, Hadi HA, Fadel HE, et al. Benign intracranial hypertension in pregnancy: current diagnostic and therapeutic approach. Obstet Gynecol Surv 1983;38:314–21.

66. Samples JR, Meyer SM. Use of ophthalmic medications in pregnant and nursing women. Am J Ophthalmol 1988;106:616–23.
67. Falardeau J, Lobb BM, Golden S, et al. The use of acetazolamide during pregnancy in intracranial hypertension patients. J Neuroophthalmol 2013;33(1):9–12.
68. Lee AG, Pless M, Falardeau J, et al. The use of acetazolamide in idiopathic intracranial hypertension during pregnancy. Am J Ophthalmol 2005;139(5):855–9.
69. Alsaad AM, Chaudhry SA, Koren G. First trimester exposure to topiramate and the risk of oral clefts in the offspring: a systematic review and meta-analysis. Reprod Toxicol 2015;53:45–50.
70. Tang RA, Dorotheo EU, Schiffman JS, et al. Medical and surgical management of idiopathic intracranial hypertension in pregnancy. Curr Neurol Neurosci Rep 2004;4:398–409.
71. Thirumalaikumar L, Ramalingam K, Heafield T. Idiopathic intracranial hypertension in pregnancy. Obstet Gynaecol 2014;16:93–7.
72. Hopkins EL, Hendricks CH, Cibils LA. Cerebrospinal fluid pressure in labor. Am J Obstet Gynecol 1965;93:907–16.
73. McCausland AM, Holmes F. Spinal fluid pressures during labor; preliminary report. West J Surg Obstet Gynecol 1957;65:220–31.
74. Coutinho JM, Zuurbier SM, Aramideh M, et al. The incidence of cerebral venous thrombosis: a cross-sectional study. Stroke 2012;43(12):3375–7.
75. Devasagayam S, Wyatt B, Leyden J, et al. Cerebral venous sinus thrombosis incidence is higher than previously thought: a retrospective population-based study. Stroke 2016;47(9):2180–2.
76. Masuhr F, Mehraein S, Einhaupl K. Cerebral venous and sinus thrombosis. J Neurol 2004;251:11–23.
77. Ferro JM, Bousser MG, Canhão P, et al. European Stroke Organization guideline for the diagnosis and treatment of cerebral venous thrombosis. Eur J Neurol 2017;24(10):1203–13.
78. Biousse V, Ameri A, Bousser MG. Isolated intracranial hypertension as the only sign of cerebral venous thrombosis. Neurology 1999;53:1537–42.
79. Srinivasan K. Cerebral venous and arterial thrombosis in pregnancy and puerperium. A study of 135 patients. Angiology 1983;34:731–46.
80. Srinivasan K. Puerperal cerebral venous and arterial thrombosis. Semin Neurol 1988;8:222–5.
81. Aguiar de Sousa D, Canhão P, Crassard I, et al. Safety of pregnancy after cerebral venous thrombosis: results of the ISCVT (International Study on Cerebral Vein and Dural Sinus Thrombosis)-2 PREGNANCY Study. Stroke 2017;48(11):3130–3.
82. Lanska DJ, Kryscio RJ. Risk factors for peripartum and postpartum stroke and intracranial venous thrombosis. Stroke 2000;31(6):1274–82.
83. Kittner SJ, Stern BJ, Feeser BR, et al. Risk factors for peripartum and postpartum stroke and intracranial venous thrombosis. Stroke 2000;31:1274–82.
84. Kim IT, Choi JB. Occlusions of branch retinal arterioles following amniotic fluid embolism. Ophthalmologica 2000;214:305–8.
85. Bodur H, Caliskan E, Anik Y, et al. Cranial thromboembolism secondary to patent foramen ovale and deep venous thrombosis after cesarean section. Gynecol Obstet Invest 2008;65:258–61.
86. James AH, Bushnell CD, Jamison MG, et al. Incidence and risk factors for stroke in pregnancy and the puerperium. Obstet Gynecol 2005;106:509–16.
87. Davie CA, O'Brien P. Stroke and pregnancy. J Neurol Neurosurg Psychiatry 2008;79:240–5.

88. Tiel Groenestege AT, Rinkel GJ, van der Bom JG, et al. The risk of aneurysmal subarachnoid hemorrhage during pregnancy, delivery, and the puerperium in the Utrecht population: case-crossover study and standardized incidence ratio estimation. Stroke 2009;40:1148–51.
89. Horton JC, Chambers WA, Lyons SL, et al. Pregnancy and the risk of hemorrhage from cerebral arteriovenous malformations. Neurosurgery 1990;27:867–71.
90. Bateman BT, Schumacher HC, Bushnell CD, et al. Intracerebral hemorrhage in pregnancy: frequency, risk factors, and outcome. Neurology 2006;67:424–9.
91. Porras JL, Yang W, Philadelphia E, et al. Hemorrhage risk of brain arteriovenous malformations during pregnancy and puerperium in a North American cohort. Stroke 2017;48:1507–13.
92. Frederick IO, Qiu C, Enquobahrie DA, et al. Lifetime prevalence and correlates of migraine among women in a pacific northwest pregnancy cohort study. Headache 2014;54(4):675–85.
93. Fox AW, Davis RL. Migraine chronobiology. Headache 1998;38(06):436–41.
94. Broner SW, Bobker S, Klebanoff L. Migraine in women. Semin Neurol 2017;37(6):601–10.
95. Aubé M. Migraine in pregnancy. Neurology 1999;53(4 Suppl 1):S26–8.
96. Jarvis DP, Piercy CN. Managing migraine in pregnancy. BMJ 2018;25:360, k80.
97. Martins LB, Rodrigues AMDS, Rodrigues DF, et al. Double-blind placebo-controlled randomized clinical trial of ginger (Zingiber officinale Rosc.) addition in migraine acute treatment. Cephalalgia 2018. https://doi.org/10.1177/0333102418776016.
98. Chen HM, Chen SF, Chen YH, et al. Increased risk of adverse pregnancy outcomes for women with migraines: a nationwide population-based study. Cephalalgia 2010;30(04):433–8.
99. Wells RE, Turner DP, Lee M, et al. Managing migraine during pregnancy and lactation. Curr Neurol Neurosci Rep 2016;16:40.
100. Tietjen GE, Collins SA. Hypercoagulability and migraine. Headache 2018;58:173–83.
101. Cohen Y, Lavie O, Granovsky-Grisaru S, et al. Bell palsy complicating pregnancy: a review. Obstet Gynecol Surv 2000;55:184–8.
102. Hussain A, Nduka C, Moth P, et al. Bell's facial nerve palsy in pregnancy: a clinical review. J Obstet Gynaecol 2017;37(4):409–15.
103. Phillips KM, Heiser A, Gaudin R, et al. Onset of bell's palsy in late pregnancy and early puerperium is associated with worse long-term outcomes. Laryngoscope 2017;127(12):2854–9.
104. Vallejo-Vaz AJ, Stiefel P, Alfaro V, et al. Isolated abducens nerve palsy in preeclampsia and hypertension in pregnancy. Hypertens Res 2013;36(9):834–5.
105. Nieto-Calvache AJ, Loaiza-Osorio S, Casallas-Carrillo J, et al. Abducens nerve palsy in gestational hypertension: a case report and review of the literature. J Obstet Gynaecol Can 2017;39(10):890–3.
106. Jacobson DM. Superior oblique palsy manifested during pregnancy. Ophthalmology 1991;98(12):1874–6.
107. Sprung J, Haddox JD, Maitra-D'Cruze AM. Horner's syndrome and trigeminal nerve palsy following epidural anaesthesia for obstetrics. Can J Anaesth 1991;38:767–71.
108. Chambers DJ, Bhatia K. Cranial nerve palsy following central neuraxial block in obstetrics: a review of the literature and analysis of 43 case reports. Int J Obstet Anesth 2017;31:13–26.

109. Muthyala T, Bagga R, Saha SC, et al. Isolated oculomotor nerve palsy with complete recovery in eclampsia: a rare presentation. J Obstet Gynaecol 2016;36(7): 848–9.

110. Gilca M, Luneau K. Multiple concomitant cranial nerve palsies secondary to preeclampsia. J Neuroophthalmol 2015;35(2):179–81.

111. Digre KB, Varner MW, Schiffman JS. Neuroophthalmologic effects of intravenous magnesium sulfate. Am J Obstet Gynecol 1990;163:1848–52.

112. Folk JC, Weingeist TA. Fundus changes in toxaemia. Ophthalmology 1981;88: 1173–4.

113. Beck RW, Gamel JW, Willcourt RJ, et al. Acute ischemic optic neuropathy in severe preeclampsia. Am J Ophthalmol 1980;90(3):342–6.

114. Giridhar P, Freedman K. Nonarteritic anterior ischemic optic neuropathy in a 35-year-old postpartum woman with recent preeclampsia. JAMA Ophthalmol 2013; 131(4):542–4.

115. Watson DL, Sibai BM, Shaver DC, et al. Late postpartum eclampsia: an update. South Med J 1983;76:1487–9.

116. Sabet HY, Blake P, Nguyen D. Alexia without agraphia in a postpartum eclamptic patient with factor V Leiden deficiency. AJNR Am J Neuroradiol 2004;25:419–20.

117. Imes RK, Kutzscher E, Gardner R. Binasal hemianopias from presumed intrageniculate myelinolysis: report of a case with MR images of bilateral geniculate involvement after emergency cesarean section and hysterectomy. Neuroophthalmology 2002;28:45–50.

118. Chien PF, Khan KS, Arnott N. Magnesium sulphate in the treatment of eclampsia and pre-eclampsia: an overview of the evidence from randomised trials. Br J Obstet Gynaecol 1996;103:1085–91.

119. Euser AG, Cipolla MJ. Magnesium sulfate for the treatment of eclampsia: a brief review. Stroke 2009;40(4):1169–75.

120. Kanal E, Barkovich AJ, Bell C, et al. ACR guidance document for safe MR practices. AJR Am J Roentgenol 2007;188:1447–74.

121. Committee on Obstetric Practice. Committee Opinion No. 723: guidelines for diagnostic imaging during pregnancy and lactation. Obstet Gynecol 2017; 130:e210–6.

122. Wang PI, Chong ST, Kielar AZ, et al. Imaging of pregnant and lactating patients: part 1, evidence-based review and recommendations. AJR Am J Roentgenol 2012;198:778–84.

123. Greenberg F, Lewis RA. Safety of fluorescein angiography during pregnancy. Am J Ophthalmol 1990;110:323–5.

124. Fineman MS, Maguire JI, Fineman SW, et al. Safety of indocyanine green angiography during pregnancy: a survey of the retina, macula, and vitreous societies. Arch Ophthalmol 2001;119:353–5.

125. Rubinchik-Sterna M, Shmuela M, Barb J, et al. Maternal–fetal transfer of indocyanine green across the perfused human placenta. Reprod Toxicol 2016;62: 100–5.

Lower Extremity Weakness and Numbness in the Postpartum Period

A Case-Based Review

Mary Angela O'Neal, MD

KEYWORDS

- Lower extremity • Compression neuropathy • Postpartum • Neuraxial anesthesia

KEY POINTS

- In the postpartum period, consultations for lower extremity pain, weakness, numbness, and sphincter disturbances are common.
- The etiology of the lower extremity symptoms is commonly due to a compression neuropathy and rarely caused by the anesthetic technique.
- Compression neuropathies are usually caused by focal demyelination and have an excellent prognosis.

INCIDENCE

Postpartum obstetric neuropathies occur in approximately 1% of deliveries.[1] The incidence of injury in descending order of risk is the lateral cutaneous femoral, femoral, fibular, lumbosacral plexus, sciatic, and obturator nerves.[1] In contrast, complications related to either epidural or spinal anesthesia, neuraxial procedures, are rare. Reported estimates of adverse events related to epidural anesthesia after combining multiple studies are as follows: risk of an epidural hematoma, 1 in 168,000, and risk of an epidural infection, 1 in 145,000.[2]

RISK FACTORS

Risk factors for developing a postpartum lower extremity neuropathy include short stature, nulliparity, excessive weight gain, fetal macrosomia, or malpresentation. Additional risk factors include instrumental delivery and a prolonged second stage of labor.

Disclosure Statement: The author has no disclosures of financial conflict of interest. The author received no funding for this endeavor.

Department of Neurology, Brigham and Women's Hospital, 60 Fenwood Road, Boston, MA 02115, USA

E-mail address: maoneal@bwh.harvard.edu

Neurol Clin 37 (2019) 103–111
https://doi.org/10.1016/j.ncl.2018.09.002
0733-8619/19/© 2018 Elsevier Inc. All rights reserved.

Neuraxial anesthesia also increases the risk of an obstetric neuropathy because the lack of sensation contributes to decreased repositioning.[1,3]

PROGNOSIS

The overall prognosis for postpartum neuropathies is excellent, because the injury is typically related to stretch or compression leading to focal demyelination. The expected recovery time is usually 6 to 8 weeks. The presence of any underlying neuropathy confers a worse prognosis because there is more likely to be additional axonal injury.

LATERAL FEMORAL CUTANEOUS NERVE
Case 1

A 38-year-old G1P1* comes in for evaluation of numbness in her leg, which she developed after giving birth. She noted that her left thigh felt numb when she shaved her legs. She denied any pain or leg weakness.

On examination, she had a normal neurologic examination except for an area of numbness over her left lateral thigh that respected the midline.

*G, gravida (the number of pregnancies); P, parity (the number of pregnancies carried to a viable gestational age).

Anatomy and clinical findings
The lateral femoral cutaneous nerve is the most common lower extremity neuropathy. Its incidence is 0.4%.[4] The nerve is formed from the dorsal roots of L2 to L3. It courses lateral to the psoas muscle, crosses the illiacus muscle, and then goes under the inguinal ligament to supply sensation to the lateral thigh. The nerve has no motor component. The clinical findings of loss of sensation over the lateral thigh which respects the midline are pathognomonic. There may or may not be associated pain– meralgia paresthetica and a Tinel's sign may be present at the inguinal ligament (the phenomena where tapping over an area where a nerve is injured causes pain and/or paresthesia in the distribution of that nerve).

Etiology
Risk factors to develop this neuropathy include obesity, diabetes, and pregnancy. In pregnancy, the nerve can be compressed as it courses under the inguinal ligament by excessive weight gain, edema, a large fetus, or prolonged pushing in the lithotomy position.[5]

Treatment
Treatment is aimed at pain control. In the postpartum setting, a local lidocaine (Lidoderm) patch can be very effective.[6] Nonsteroidal antiinflammatory medications are also safe and occasionally efficacious. The usual medications used to treat neuropathic pain are effective, many of which are compatible with breast feeding (**Table 1**).

FEMORAL NERVE
Case 2

A 34-year-old G1P1 woman with a history of gestational diabetes delivered a 5-lb, 8-oz baby. An uncomplicated epidural was placed for labor analgesia. She had 3 hours of second stage labor and required vacuum assistance to deliver. While she was pushing, her legs felt numb. Later, she found that both legs were weak, the right more than the left. She reported numbness in her anterior thighs and below her knees, which was more pronounced on the right. There was no pain or sphincter disturbance.

Table 1 Medications used for neuropathic pain		
Medication Name	**Pregnancy Risk Category**	**Breastfeeding Risk**
Pregabalin	C	Unknown
Gabapentin	C	Excreted into breast milk No reported adverse newborn outcomes
Duloxetine	C	Not recommended
Tricyclic antidepressants	C	Not recommended
Carbamazepine	D	Compatible

From O'Neal MA, Chang LY, Salajegheh MK. Postpartum spinal cord, root, plexus and peripheral nerve injuries involving the lower extremities: a practical approach. Anesth Analg 2015;120(1):141–8; with permission.

On examination, she was 5 feet 6 inches tall and weighed 125 pounds. Lower extremity motor examination showed strength of 4 of 5 for the right hip flexors and 3 of 5 for the right knee extensors. The rest of her strength was full, including hip abductors and adductors. Her reflexes were remarkable for absent knee jerks bilaterally and diminished pinprick over the right thigh and anterior shin. Her gait was remarkable for the proximal weakness on the right.

The patient was diagnosed with bilateral femoral neuropathies.

Anatomy and clinical findings

The incidence of femoral neuropathy is 2.8 in 100,000 with up to one-quarter of the cases being bilateral, as in the vignette presented.[7,8] The femoral nerve is derived from the L2 to L3 roots. The nerve descends from the lumbar plexus traveling lateral to the psoas muscle. It passes under approximately the midpoint of the inguinal ligament. It innervates the thigh muscles that flex the hip joint and extend the knee as well as supplies sensation to the anteromedial thigh (anterior cutaneous branches of the femoral nerve) and the medial side of the leg and foot (saphenous nerve).

Patients who have a femoral neuropathy complain of difficulty standing from a sitting position. On examination, patients may have weakness in the hip flexors and quadriceps muscles, loss of the ipsilateral patellar reflex, and sensory loss in the medial thigh and calf. They may also have associated neuropathic pain.

Etiology

The nerve is generally compressed owing to excessive hip abduction, a large fetus, prolonged lithotomy position, and instrumental vaginal delivery.[8] It is most commonly compressed at the inguinal ligament, but can also be compromised in the retroperitoneum by hemorrhage or intrapelvic pathology (**Fig. 1**). It is often difficult to distinguish a femoral neuropathy from an L2 to L3 radiculopathy or an upper lumbar plexopathy. Thus, imaging and electrodiagnostic testing may be necessary.

Treatment

Treatment is composed of physical therapy to maximize motor function. A brace is often needed to stabilize the knee to prevent buckling owing to quadriceps weakness. Medications and nerve blocks are used to treat neuropathic pain.

Pelvic Nerves

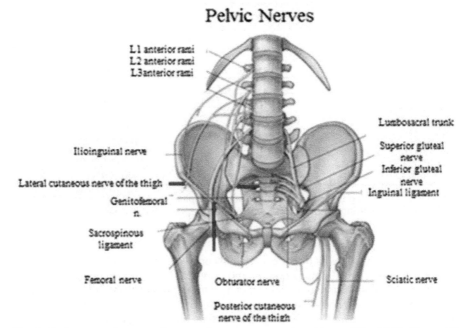

L1 anterior rami
L2 anterior rami
L3anterior rami

Lumbosacral trunk

Superior gluteal nerve
Inferior gluteal nerve
Inguinal ligament

Ilioinguinal nerve

Lateral cutaneous nerve of the thigh

Genitofemoral n.

Sacrospinous ligament

Femoral nerve

Obturator nerve

Sciatic nerve

Posterior cutaneous nerve of the thigh

Fig. 1. Red arrows show usual areas of nerve compression. (*From* O'Neal MA, Chang LY, Salajegheh MK. Postpartum spinal cord, root, plexus and peripheral nerve injuries involving the lower extremities: a practical approach. Anesth Analg 2015;120(1):141–8; with permission.)

FIBULAR NERVE
Case 3

A 32-year-old, right-handed woman 8 weeks postpartum was evaluated for left leg pain, numbness, and weakness, which she thought was related to her epidural anesthesia. She had an uneventful initiation of epidural labor analgesia, but eventually required a cesarean delivery for nonreassuring fetal status during the second stage of labor. Postpartum, she developed left leg pain and paresthesia, as well as weakness of her left leg below the knee. Her symptoms were aggravated by crossing her legs. She had mild back pain without radicular pain.

On examination, she had full back range of motion without pain and a negative straight leg raising test (a maneuver that stretches the sciatic nerve). She had 4 out of 5 weakness involving the left anterior tibialis and extensor halluces muscles, as well as mild left foot evertor weakness. She had full strength in the remaining lower extremity muscles, including foot invertors and plantar flexors. Her reflexes were normal. There was a positive Tinel's sign over the fibular nerve at the head of the fibular bone. The rest of her sensory examination was normal. Her gait was notable for a left foot drop with associated difficulty standing on her left heel.

Anatomy and clinical findings
The fibular nerve supplies sensation to the lateral calf and dorsum of the foot. It also supplies motor innervation to the foot dorsiflexors and evertors, leading to a foot drop. Patients develop a steppage gait to overcome the foot drop.

Etiology

The nerve is most commonly injured at the fibular head, where it lies in a superficial location. Injury is often bilateral. In labor, it is commonly injured by prolonged squatting or owing to hand positioning holding the legs.[9–12]

Treatment

Physical therapy is important to teach the patient how to compensate for the foot drop and prevent falls, especially while carrying an infant. In addition, an ankle foot orthotic brace is often required to minimize the foot drop.

LUMBOSACRAL PLEXOPATHY

Anatomy and Clinical Findings

The first 4 lumbar roots form the lumbar plexus. The major nerves formed from the lumbar plexus include the ilioinguinal, iliohypogastric, genitofemoral, lateral femoral cutaneous, femoral, and obturator nerves. These nerves supply the motor function to the anterior and medial thigh and involve sensation in the groin, mons pubis, labia majora, lateral gluteal, lateral thigh, and medial leg.

Portions of the fourth and fifth lumbar roots and the first 3 sacral roots form the sacral plexus. The superior and inferior gluteal nerves come directly off the plexus to supply the gluteus medius and maximus. The sciatic and the pudendal nerves are the other main nerves derived from the sacral plexus. The pudendal nerve is responsible for the somatic innervation of the sphincters and perineum.

A lumbosacral plexopathy presents in a similar fashion as a polyradiculopathy, but without back pain. Owing to the overlap, imaging of both the lumbar spine and plexus are often needed. An electromyogram/nerve conduction study can be helpful to distinguish the 2 entities by showing a lack of paraspinal denervation in a plexopathy.[13]

Etiology

The most common postpartum causes of a lumbar plexopathy are due to labor positioning, compression by the fetus, or injury from an instrumental delivery. The pelvic brim is the usual site of compression.[14]

Treatment

Treatment involves appropriate bracing for quadriceps weakness and physical therapy. Medications are also often needed to treat neuropathic pain.

SCIATIC NERVE

Case 4

A 36-year-old woman, G1P1, was evaluated for left leg pain that had started during pregnancy, but worsened postpartum. She described severe pain in the left buttocks that radiated down the lateral aspect of her leg to the top of the foot. The pain was burning and aggravated by sitting. There was associated numbness. She denied back pain, leg weakness, or any sphincter disturbance.

On examination, she had full lower extremity strength with normal reflexes. Her sensation was preserved to all modalities. There was a positive straight leg raising sign at 30° on the left. To palpation, there was significant tenderness over her left buttock, but no back tenderness. She was diagnosed with a piriformis syndrome causing sciatic nerve dysfunction.

Anatomy and clinical findings

Sciatic nerve injuries happen infrequently postpartum. One retrospective review found the incidence to be 2 in 6046 births.[1] The sciatic nerve is 2 nerves encased together, the fibular and posterior tibial nerves. In addition to a foot drop and weakness of ankle evertors, there should also be invertor ankle weakness. There may be plantar flexor weakness, but because the gastrocnemius muscle is one of the strongest muscles, this finding is often difficult to elicit. Sensory loss involves the lateral calf and the foot, both dorsal and plantar aspects. Further, the Achilles reflex can be affected.

Etiology

As in other postpartum neuropathies, nulliparity, a prolonged second stage of labor, instrumental delivery, and a large fetus are risk factors for this compressive nerve injury. In addition, the nerve can be injured by injections into the buttocks.[15] In our case, the sciatic nerve was irritated owing to spasm of the piriformis muscle.[16–18]

Treatment

Physical therapy is the mainstay of treatment, along with an ankle foot orthotic brace if there is a foot drop. During pregnancy, local analgesics such as a lidocaine patch or pain medications may be required. Postpartum medications for neuropathic pain such as tricyclics or gabapentin may be used. Both these medications are a Hale L2 breast feeding safety category meaning that they have been studied in a limited number of women without any adverse effects on nursing infants[13] (see **Table 1**).

OBTURATOR NERVE
Anatomy and Clinical Findings

An obturator neuropathy is the least common of the lower extremity nerve injuries accounting for only 4.7% of all lower extremity nerve injuries.[1] The obturator nerve innervates the hip adductors and supplies sensation to the medial thigh. An obturator nerve injury causes a wide-based gait with circumduction because the hip abductors are unopposed.

Etiology

The obturator nerve is most commonly compressed at the posterior inferior aspect of the pelvic brim[13] (see **Fig. 1**). Risk factors for injury include instrumental vaginal delivery, cephalopelvic disproportion, and labor positioning.

Treatment

The treatment for an obturator neuropathy is physical therapy.

COMPLICATIONS OF NEURAXIAL ANESTHESIA

Neuraxial anesthesia can cause neurologic injuries involving the lower extremities. However, these injuries are much less frequent than obstetric injuries. For example, they are estimated to occur in only 12 in 1 million women.[19] The etiology of the neurologic dysfunction is diverse including direct trauma, epidural hematoma, epidural abscess, spinal block, and spinal cord ischemia. A careful evaluation is imperative to distinguish these injuries from the more usual birth trauma-related neuropathies.

Case 5

A 33-year-old woman, G3P3, presented to the neurology service for pain evaluation 2 days after a normal spontaneous vaginal delivery with epidural analgesia. When getting up from the sitting position, she noted brief electric shocklike pain from her low thoracic spine radiating upward to the occiput as well as down into her lower back (Lhermitte's phenomena owing to posterior column irritation). The patient was afebrile with stable vital signs. The patient perceived that the epidural procedure was difficult and had required multiple attempts by the anesthesiologist.

Her neurologic examination was normal. Neck flexion elicited the shocklike pain. She was not taking any anticoagulants, and her platelet count and coagulation studies were normal (**Fig. 2**). Her symptoms were related to the anesthesia technique introducing blood into the subarachnoid space.

DIRECT TRAUMA

Trauma from neuraxial anesthesia can be related to either catheter or needle injury or to the injection of local anesthetics into the nerve root, cord, or conus medullaris. The common causes of the trauma are related to a low-lying conus, high placement of the needle, or trauma related to catheter placement.[20] The neurologic syndromes that result can include radicular pain, numbness, weakness, a spinal cord syndrome or a conus medullaris syndrome–painless bowel, and bladder associated with perineal sensory loss.

EPIDURAL HEMATOMA

This is a rare complication with an incidence of 1 in 168,000 neuraxial procedures in an obstetric population.[19] It is frequently associated with patients on anticoagulants, antiplatelet drugs, or in situations where there is a coagulopathy. Epidural hematomas

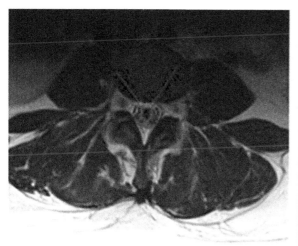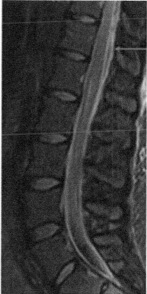

Fig. 2. Axial and sagittal T2 lumbar MRIs showing subacute blood (3–7 days old) in the subdural and subarachnoid spaces. The arrows are pointing to the dark signal, which represents methemoglobin. (*From* O'Neal MA, Chang LY, Salajegheh MK. Postpartum spinal cord, root, plexus and peripheral nerve injuries involving the lower extremities: a practical approach. Anesth Analg 2015;120(1):141–8; with permission.)

tend to occur early when the epidural catheter is in place.[21,22] If there is significant neurologic compromise the, hematoma needs to be decompressed immediately.

EPIDURAL ABSCESS

This complication is most often seen 5 to 8 days after the procedure. Patients present with fever and usually severe back pain over the involved site. The neurologic examination will depend on the extent of cord and/or root involvement. Unless there is significant neural involvement, first-line treatment is with appropriate antibiotics.

SPINAL CORD ISCHEMIA

There have been rare cases of anterior spinal artery syndromes related to neuraxial anesthesia.[23–25] The anterior spinal artery supplies the anterior two-thirds of the cord with 2 posterior spinal arteries supplying the posterior columns. The artery of Adamkiewicz is a major radicular feeder of the lower spinal cord. It arises from the aorta usually at the thoracic, T8 to L 1 levels. The clinical syndrome involves bilateral lower extremity weakness, bowel and bladder incontinence with loss of pain, and temperature sense below T12 with preservation of vibratory and joint position sense in the legs. Most cases occur in the setting of hypotension or aortic surgery. In the few cases related to neuraxial anesthesia, it is postulated that patients with vascular risk factors in the presence of sympathomimetic anesthetics there was vasoconstriction leading to cord ischemia.

TAKE HOME POINTS

- Difficulties related to lower extremity pain, weakness, numbness, and sphincter disturbances are a common cause for both neurologic and obstetric anesthesia consultations.
- The etiology of the lower extremity symptoms is commonly due to a compression neuropathy and rarely caused by the anesthetic technique.
- Compression neuropathies are usually caused by focal demyelination and have an excellent prognosis.

REFERENCES

1. Wong CA, Scavone BM, Dugan S, et al. Incidence of postpartum lumbosacral spine and lower extremity nerve injuries. Obstet Gynecol 2003;101:279–88.
2. Ruppen W, Derry S, McQuay H, et al. Incidence of epidural hematoma, infection, and neurologica injury in obstetric patients with epidural analgesia/anesthesia. Anesthesiology 2006;104:394–9.
3. Massey EW, Guidon AC. Peripheral neuropathies in pregnancy. Continuum (Minneap Minn) 2014;20(1):100–14.
4. Scott K. Neural injury during pregnancy and childbirth. Musculoskeletal health in pregnancy and postpartum. p. 93–114.
5. Van Diver T, Camann W. Meralgia paresthetica in a parturient. Int J Obstet Anesth 1995;4(2):109–12.
6. Meier T, Wasner G, Faust M, et al. Efficacy of Lidoderm patch 5% in the treatment of focal peripheral neuropathic pain syndromes: a randomized double blind, placebo-controlled study. Pain 2003;106:151–8.
7. Vargo MM, Robinson LR, Nicholas JJ, et al. Postpartum femoral neuropathy: relic of an earlier era? Arch Phys Med Rehabil 1990;71(8):591–6.

8. Massey EW, Stolp KA. Peripheral neuropathy in pregnancy. Phys Med Rehabil Clin N Am 2008;19:149–62.
9. Radawski MM, Strakowski JA, Johnson EW. Acute common peroneal neuropathy due to hand positioning in normal labor and delivery. Obstet Gynecol 2011;118: 421–3.
10. Adornato BT, Carlini WG. "Pushing palsy' a case of self-induced bilateral peroneal palsy during natural childbirth. Neurology 1992;42:936–7
11. Reif ME. Bilateral common peroneal nerve palsy secondary to prolonged squatting in natural childbirth. Birth 1988;15:100–2.
12. Babayev M, Bodack MP, Creatura C. Common peroneal neuropathy secondary to squatting during childbirth. Obstet Gynecol 1998;91:830–2.
13. O'Neal MA, Chang LY, Salajegheh MK. Postpartum spinal cord, root, plexus and peripheral nerve injuries involving the lower extremities: a practical approach. Anesth Analg 2015;120:141–8.
14. Feasby TE, Burton SR, Hahn AF. Obstetrical lumbosacral plexus injury. Muscle Nerve 1992;15:937–40.
15. Kim HJ, Park SH. Sciatic nerve injection injury. J Int Med Res 2014;42(4):887–97.
16. Vallejo MC, Mariano DJ, Kaul B, et al. Piriformis syndrome in a patient after cesarean section under spinal anesthesia. Reg Anesth Pain Med 2004;29(4):364–7.
17. Sivrioglu AK, Ozyurek S, Mutlu H, et al. Piriformis syndrome occurring after pregnancy. BMJ Case Rep 2013. https://doi.org/10.1136/bcr-2013-008946.
18. Papadopoulos EC, Khan SN. Piriformis syndrome and low back pain: a new classification and review of the literature. Orthop Clin North Am 2004;35(1):65–71.
19. Ruppen W, Derry S, McQuay H, et al. Incidence of epidural hematoma, infection, and neurologic injury in obstetric patients with epidural analgesia/anesthesia. Anesthesiology 2006;105:394–9.
20. Kowe O, Waters JH. Neurologic complications in the patient receiving obstetric anesthesia. Neurol Clin 2012;30:823–33.
21. Christie IW, McCabe S. Major complications of epidural analgesia after surgery: results of a six-year survey. Anaesthesia 2007;62:335–41.
22. Okano K, Kondo H, Tsuchiya R, et al. Spinal epidural abscess associated with epidural catheterization: report of a case and a review of the literature. Jpn J Clin Oncol 1999;29:49–52.
23. Eastwood DW. Anterior spinal artery syndrome after epidural anesthesia in a pregnant diabetic patient with scleredema. Anesth Analg 1991;73(1):90–1.
24. Gong J, Gao H, Gao Y, et al. Anterior spinal artery syndrome after spinal anaesthesia for caesarean delivery with normal lumbar and thoracic magnetic resonance imaging. J Obstet Gynaecol 2016;36(7):1–2.
25. Yoshida S, Nitta Y, Oda K. Anterior spinal artery syndrome after minimally invasive direct coronary artery bypass grafting under general combined epidural anesthesia. Jpn J Thorac Cardiovasc Surg 2005;53(4):230–3.

Management of Myasthenia Gravis in Pregnancy

Janet Waters, MD, MBA

KEYWORDS

- Myasthenia gravis • Pregnancy • Neonatal myasthenia gravis • Magnesium
- Preeclampsia/eclampsia • Thymectomy • Arthrogryposis

KEY POINTS

- Myasthenia gravis is an autoimmune disorder characterized by fluctuating weakness of extraocular and proximal limb muscles, which often presents in women during childbearing years.
- Among pregnant women with myasthenia gravis, 40% have worsening symptoms during pregnancy and 20% require ventilatory support.
- In children born to women with myasthenia gravis, there is a 10% to 20% risk of developing transient neonatal myasthenia gravis.
- Vaginal delivery and epidural anesthesia are not contraindicated.
- Although pregnancy can increase the risk of worsening symptoms in the short term, there are no long-term adverse effects on the disease.

INTRODUCTION

Myasthenia gravis is an autoimmune disorder characterized by fluctuating weakness of extraocular and proximal limb muscles. In severe cases, involvement of respiratory muscles may occur. It occurs in 1 in 5000 in the overall population[1] and it is 2 times more common in women than in men. The onset in women is most common in the third decade, and risk of severe exacerbation occurs most frequently in the first year after presentation. The disease does not have an impact on fertility, and overlap with pregnancy is expected.[2] This article provides a description of the disease process and its impact on the expecting mother, fetus, and newborn child. Management options in pregnancy and lactation are discussed in detail.

PATHOGENESIS

Myasthenia is the Greek word for muscle weakness. It comes in several forms, including an acquired disorder (most common), a hereditary disorder, and transient

Women's Neurology, University of Pittsburgh Medical Center, 3471 Fifth Avenue Suite 810, Pittsburgh, PA 15213, USA
E-mail address: watersjf@upmc.edu

Neurol Clin 37 (2019) 113–120
https://doi.org/10.1016/j.ncl.2018.09.003
0733-8619/19/© 2018 Elsevier Inc. All rights reserved.

neurologic.theclinics.com

neonatal myasthenia gravis, which affects infants born to mothers with the disease.[3] Acquired myasthenia gravis is an autoimmune disorder in which antibodies block the receptor sites in striated muscle, preventing the transmission of impulses through the muscle that lead to contraction. The pathogenesis of myasthenia gravis involves both humeral and cell-mediated immunity.[2]

Patients with the disease have immunoglobulin G (IgG) antibodies that adhere to the acetylcholine receptor (AChR) in the postsynaptic junction. The production of anti-AChR antibodies is modulated by CD4 helper T cells. Autoantibodies seem to accelerate degradation and endocytosis of the AChR.[4–6] Muscles affected by myasthenia gravis have a 70% to 89% reduction in the number of AChRs per neuromuscular junction.[7]

AChR antibodies are detectable in the serum of 80% to 90% of people with generalized myasthenia gravis. Those whose disease is limited to oculomotor dysfunction may be seropositive at a much lower rate of 50%.[8] Individuals who are found seronegative for AChR antibodies may be tested for the muscle-specific kinase (MuSK); 40% of seronegative patients with clinical evidence of myasthenia gravis are found to have anti-MuSK antibodies. This subset occurs more commonly in women and produces prominent bulbar, neck, shoulder girdle and respiratory muscle weakness.[9]

Thymic hyperplasia is found in 60% to 80% of patients with acquired myasthenia gravis, and thymoma is found in 21%.[10] It is not uncommon for individuals with acquired myasthenia gravis to have other concurrent autoimmune disorders, including thyroid disease.

Patients with fatigable weakness have been described as far back as 1600. In the 1930s, the first anticholinesterase agents were introduced, including physostigmine, neostigmine, and pyridostigmine. These agents block acetylcholinesterase, an enzyme that breaks down acetylcholine. This leads to higher levels of acetylcholine at the neuromuscular junction, which augments neuromuscular transmission.

CLINICAL PRESENTATION

Myasthenia gravis often presents with ocular symptoms with double vision, disconjugate gaze, and ptosis. Ptosis is enhanced with prolonged upward gaze and double vision is not present if 1 eye is closed; 85% of these individuals progress to involve limb muscles within 3 years of onset.[1,2,7] Generalized symptoms involve proximal upper or lower extremity weakness, which worsens with repetitive activity. Patients may complain of difficulty climbing stairs or brushing their hair. Symptoms tend to progress toward the end of the day. Approximately 15% of patients develop bulbar symptoms, including dysphagia, dysarthria, and facial and neck muscle weakness. There is no associated sensory loss or ataxia and reflexes remain intact. There may be periods of spontaneous remission. Stressors, such as infection and surgery, may trigger disease progression. Several drugs can precipitate an exacerbation of symptoms and are listed in **Box 1**. Myasthenic crisis is defined as weakness of respiratory muscles that is severe enough to require intubation and ventilatory assistance. Myasthenic crises and fatalities are most frequent within 2 years to 3 years of presentation.[11]

THYMECTOMY

Thymectomy can result in complete remission in disease in 40% to 50% of patients and has become the standard of care.[3] Noncontrast chest CT is the is the preferred form of imaging in the general population. Iodinated contrast has been reported to trigger exacerbation of myasthenia gravis symptoms. Noncontrast MRI may be used safely in the pregnant population to assess for thymoma or thymic hyperplasia

---

Box 1
Medications known to exacerbate symptoms of myasthenia gravis

Marked contraindications
  D-Penicillamine and α-interferon cause increased weakness and should not be used in patients with myasthenia gravis.

Relative contraindications; avoid if possible
- Succinylcholine, D-tubocurarine, vecuronium, and other neuromuscular blocking agents, including botulinum toxins
- Quinine, quinidine, and procainamide
- β-Blockers, including propranolol, atenolol, and timolol maleate eye drops
- Calcium channel blockers
- Iodinated contrast agents
- Magnesium, including milk of magnesia, antacids containing magnesium hydroxide, and magnesium sulfate
- Select antibiotics including
  o Aminoglycosides (eg, tobramycin, gentamycin, kanamycin, neomycin, and streptomycin)
  o Macrolides(eg, erythromycin, azithromycin, and telithromycin)
  o Colistin

---

but does not visualize the anterior mediastinum as well as CT. Thymoma is uncommon in younger patients, particularly if they are seronegative.[12,13] It is reasonable to delay CT until after delivery in pregnant patients, particularly those who are seronegative.[14] Women who undergo thymectomy prior to conception have a lower incidence of disease exacerbation[15] and offspring have a lower risk of neonatal myasthenia gravis.[16] Thymectomy prior to conception is advisable.

EFFECTS OF PREGNANCY ON MYASTHENIA GRAVIS

The effects of pregnancy on myasthenia gravis are variable from woman to woman and from pregnancy to pregnancy in the same individual. A large case series done in 1999 revealed that 41% of women had worsening of symptoms during pregnancy, 29% improved, and 30% remained unchanged.[17] Disease exacerbation is more likely in the first trimester and the postpartum period. The physiologic changes of early pregnancy, including emesis, increased blood volume, and decreased gastrointestinal absorption, may increase dosage requirements for medication; 20% of women with myasthenia gravis require ventilatory assistance during pregnancy and the postpartum period. Exacerbations may occur in pregnancy regardless of the level of control prior to conception. Pregnancy termination has not been found beneficial.[3] In the long term, pregnancy does not have an adverse effect on the disease. Because myasthenic crisis and mortality tend to occur within the first 1 year to 2 years after diagnosis as well as in early pregnancy and the postpartum period, delaying pregnancy until after the first 1 year to 2 years of presentation is widely advocated.[17]

EFFECTS OF MYASTHENIA GRAVIS ON PREGNANCY AND DELIVERY

Myasthenia gravis does not increase the risk of miscarriage or preeclampsia/eclampsia. During pregnancy, the diaphragm becomes progressively elevated, increased participation by intercostal muscles to meet increase respiratory demands. Careful monitoring of respiratory status in pregnancy is necessary.[3] Myasthenia gravis may be a factor in causing spontaneous preterm birth in the setting of congenital myasthenia, discussed later.

EFFECTS OF MYASTHENIA GRAVIS ON THE FETUS

In pregnancy, maternal IgG antibodies cross the placenta and provide the newborn with a full host of immunity for the first weeks of life. In patients with myasthenia gravis, this transfer can result in transient neonatal myasthenia in 10% to 20% of newborns. Onset of symptoms may be delayed for 12 hours to several days in the offspring of women treated with water soluble anticholinesterase agents prior to delivery. Affected babies may develop decreased muscle tone, poor sucking, ptosis, and respiratory difficulties. Offspring of mothers with myasthenia gravis require close observation after delivery. There is no correlation between the severity of the mother's symptoms and the occurrence of neonatal myasthenia gravis.[18–20] In a majority of infants, degradation of maternal antibodies take place and spontaneous recovery occurs in 3 weeks to 4 weeks.

In some infants, a more severe and potentially fatal form of congenital myasthenia may occur. It occurs more often in the offspring of mothers who generate antibodies against fetal AChR rather than the more common adult AChR. It causes fetal movement dysfunction early in the pregnancy, resulting in polyhydramnios and joint contractures due to arthrogryposis multiplex. Spontaneous premature labor can occur due to early membrane rupture.[21]

MEDICAL MANAGEMENT OF MYASTHENIA GRAVIS IN PREGNANCY AND DELIVERY

Medical management aims to improve muscle function by increasing acetylcholine levels at the neuromuscular junction and by suppressing autoantibody production. When weakness is mild, no treatment may be needed. For symptomatic relief, pyridostigmine can be safely used in recommended doses during pregnancy. Changes in gastrointestinal absorption, emesis, and physiologic changes of pregnancy may necessitate adjustment of dosage. High doses of pyridostigmine have been reported to cause uterine contractions and premature labor.[14] Corticosteroids are reasonably safe in pregnancy although there has been an association with cleft palate in first-trimester exposure and high doses have been associated with premature rupture of membrane. Intravenous immunoglobulin (IVIG) has been widely used in pregnancy for autoimmune disorders and is recommended for treatment of severe exacerbations of myasthenia gravis. Plasma exchange is another option for treatment of myasthenic crisis, but the risk of hypotension during treatment makes this a less optimal treatment in pregnancy. Azathioprine and mycophenolate mofetil are used to treat myasthenia gravis in the general population but are category D in pregnancy due to teratogenicity. Methotrexate is category X due to risk of induction of spontaneous abortion. Although rituximab and cyclosporine are listed as category C in pregnancy, they are associated with B-cell lymphocytopenia and low birth weight for gestational age, respectively (**Table 1**).

Women with myasthenia gravis in pregnancy ideally should be followed by multiple specialists with coordination of care between obstetrics, neurology, anesthesiology, pulmonology, neonatology, and intensivists when necessary. Patients should be educated in the signs and symptoms of exacerbation of the disease. Adjustment of medications should be made as needed. Baseline pulmonary function tests should be obtained as well as thyroid studies to assess for concomitant autoimmune disease. Adequate rest should be encouraged and infection treated promptly with antibiotics, which are safe in patients with myasthenia gravis (see **Box 1**). Fetal ultrasound should be carried out during the latter half of the pregnancy to assess fetal movements, breathing, and amniotic fluid.

Table 1
Therapeutic interventions in myasthenia gravis

Intervention	Side Effects	Food and Drug Administration Pregnancy Category	Teratogenicity
Pyridostigmine	Diarrhea, muscle cramps, cough with increased mucus, and bradycardia	C	Probably safe; no controlled studies
Prednisone	Weight gain, hyperglycemia, hypertension, mood changes, osteoporosis, and myopathy	C	Increased risk of cleft palate in animal studies; can be used in pregnancy
Plasma exchange	Hypercoagulability, hypotension, tachycardia, electrolyte imbalances, sepsis, allergic reaction, nausea, and vomiting	N/A	Plasma exchange has been used successfully during pregnancy.
Immunoglobulins	Hypercoagulability, headache, aseptic meningitis dermatitis, pulmonary edema, and allergic/anaphylactic reactions	C	IVIG has been used successfully during human pregnancy.
Rituximab	Fever, headache, abdominal pain, hypotension, thrombocytopenia, and progressive multifocal encephalopathy	C	B-cell lymphocytopenia generally lasting <6 mo can occur in infants exposed to rituximab in utero
Cyclosporine	Renal toxicity, hypertension, seizures, myopathy, and increased risk of infections	C	Human studies demonstrate evidence of premature birth and low birth weight for gestational age
Mycophenolate mofetil	Increased risk of infection; possible increased risk of lymphoma and skin cancer	D	Pregnancy loss in first trimester and congenital malformations in the face and distal limbs, heart, esophagus, and kidney have been reported.
Azathioprine	Hepatoxicity, bone marrow suppression, nausea, vomiting, diarrhea, and possible increased and risk of lymphoma and leukemia	D	Congenital defects, including cerebral palsy, cardiovascular defects, hypcspadias, cerebral hemorrhage, polydactyly, ard hypothyroidism

MANAGEMENT OF MYASTHENIA GRAVIS IN DELIVERY

Myometrial muscle is composed of smooth muscle and function is not affected by myasthenia gravis. The first stage of labor may proceed without intervention and cesarean section should be reserved for obstetric considerations. In the second stage of labor, striated muscles are used to augment expulsion and use of forceps or vacuum for assisted delivery may be indicated. Medication should be administered throughout the delivery to optimize voluntary muscle function.

There is no contraindication to use of epidural anesthesia during labor and delivery. Epidural anesthesia should not be allowed to rise above the T10 level to avoid compromise of respiratory muscle function. Ester-type medications, such as chloroprocaine and tetracaine, should be avoided because they may trigger worsening of muscle weakness. Amide-type medications, including lidocaine, bupivacaine, and mepivacaine, are preferable. Opioids and general anesthetics should be avoided when possible due to risk of potentiating AChR antibody effects.[3]

PREECLAMPSIA AND ECLAMPSIA IN THE MYASTHENIC PATIENT

Use of magnesium in the treatment of preeclampsia and eclampsia should be avoided in the myasthenic patient if possible. Magnesium blocks calcium entry at the nerve terminal and inhibits acetylcholine release. This can lead to a dramatic increase in muscle weakness. To protect against seizure activity, intravenous levetiracetam may be given. Phenytoin can cause increased muscle weakness in patients with myasthenia gravis.

MYASTHENIA GRAVIS IN THE POSTPARTUM PATIENT

Symptoms of myasthenia gravis can acutely worsen in the postpartum period, and deterioration can be rapid and dramatic. It can occur despite a relatively symptom-free pregnancy and close monitoring of the mother's neurologic and respiratory status is indicated. The care for a newborn can also carry challenges, including reduced sleep, frequent feedings, and the physical exertion of child care. Engagement of a support system should be encouraged.

LACTATION

The American Academy of Pediatrics considers use of prednisone, prednisolone, and pyridostigmine to be safe during lactation.[22] Cyclosporine, methotrexate, and azathioprine are considered contraindicated in lactation due to risk of immunosuppression, neutropenia, growth retardation, and potential for carcinogenesis. There are few data available to assess the safety of mycophenolate, mofetil and rituximab during lactation.

CONTRACEPTION

There have been reported cases of exacerbation of myasthenia gravis symptoms during the cyclic withdrawal of oral contraceptives.[23,24] Continuous hormonal contraceptive in the form of implant, ring, or oral contraceptive may be preferable. An intrauterine device also is a reasonable and effective alternative.

PRECONCEPTUAL COUNSELING

Ideally, a patient with myasthenia gravis presents for counseling about her disease prior to conception. She should be advised that 40% of women have worsening symptoms during pregnancy and that 20% require ventilatory support, 30% of women have improvement in their symptoms during pregnancy, and 30% see no change. Exacerbations during pregnancy tend to occur in the first trimester and postpartum period. It is safe to use pyridostigmine during pregnancy, and steroids and IVIG are safe in pregnancy should an exacerbation take place. Women who have recently been diagnosed with myasthenia gravis have the highest risk of severe exacerbation and should be advised to delay pregnancy for 1 year to 2 years after presentation. The patient should be informed that there is a 10% to 20% risk that her infant will develop transient neonatal myasthenia gravis and may require medication and other support measures for the first few weeks of life. Rarely, infants may develop severe effects from exposure to fetal IGG antibodies that can result in poor motility, joint deformities, and premature birth. The patient may be informed that vaginal delivery is not contraindicated but that assisted delivery with vacuum or forceps may be required during the second stage of delivery. Epidural anesthesia is not contraindicated. General anesthetics and opioids should be avoided if possible due to risk of worsening symptoms. Breast feeding while taking pyridostigmine or steroids is safe but may be inadvisable when taking other immunosuppressive agents. Although pregnancy can increase risk of worsening of symptoms in the short term, there are no long-term adverse effects on the disease. When discontinuing immunosuppressive therapy prior to a planned conception, contraception should be used for 6 months prior to attempting pregnancy.

REFERENCES

1. Mays J, Butts CL. Intercommunication between the neuroendocrine and immune systems: focus on myasthenia gravis. Neuroimmunomodulation 2011;18(5): 320–7.
2. Drachman DB. Myasthenia gravis. N Engl J Med 1994;330(25):1797–810.
3. Varner M. Myasthenia gravis and pregnancy. Clin Obstet Gynecol 2013;56(2): 372–81.
4. Tzartos SJ, Cung MT, Demange P, et al. The main immunogenic region (MIR) of the nicotinic acetylcholine receptor and the anti-MIR antibodies. Mol Neurobiol 1991;5(1):1–29.
5. Link H, Olsson O, Sun J, et al. Acetylcholine receptor-reactive T and B cells in myasthenia gravis and controls. J Clin Invest 1991;87(6):2191–6.
6. Appel SH, Anwyl R, McAdams MW, et al. Accelerated degradation of acetylcholine receptor from cultured rat myotubes with myasthenia gravis sera and globulins. Proc Natl Acad Sci U S A 1977;74(5):2130–4.
7. Stafford IP, Dildy GA. Myasthenia gravis and pregnancy. Clin Obstet Gynecol 2005;48(1):48–56.
8. Lindstrom JM, Seybold ME, Lennon VA, et al. Antibody to acetylcholine receptor in myasthenia gravis. Prevalence, clinical correlates, and diagnostic value. Neurology 1976;26(11):1054–9.
9. Evoli A, Tonali PA, Padua L, et al. Clinical correlates with anti-MuSK antibodies in generalized seronegative myasthenia gravis. Brain 2003;126(Pt 10):2304–11.
10. Leite MI, Strobel P, Jones M, et al. Fewer thymic changes in MuSK antibody-positive than in MuSK antibody-negative MG. Ann Neurol 2005;57(3):444–8.
11. Spring PJ, Spies JM. Myasthenia gravis: options and timing of immunomodulatory treatment. BioDrugs 2001;15(3):173–83.
12. Maggi L, Andreetta F, Antozzi C, et al. Two cases of thymoma-associated myasthenia gravis without antibodies to the acetylcholine receptor. Neuromuscul Disord 2008;18(8):678–80.

13. Choi Decroos E, Hobson-Webb LD, Juel VC, et al. Do acetylcholine receptor and striated muscle antibodies predict the presence of thymoma in patients with myasthenia gravis? Muscle Nerve 2014;49(1):30–4.
14. Massey JM, De Jesus-Acosta C. Pregnancy and myasthenia gravis. Continuum (Minneap Minn) 2014;20(1 Neurology of Pregnancy):115–27.
15. Niks EH, Verrips A, Semmekrot BA, et al. A transient neonatal myasthenic syndrome with anti-musk antibodies. Neurology 2008;70(14):1215–6.
16. Ahlsten G, Lefvert AK, Osterman PO, et al. Follow-up study of muscle function in children of mothers with myasthenia gravis during pregnancy. J Child Neurol 1992;7(3):264–9.
17. Batocchi AP, Majolini L, Evoli A, et al. Course and treatment of myasthenia gravis during pregnancy. Neurology 1999;52(3):447–52.
18. Servais L, Baudoin H, Zehrouni K, et al. Pregnancy in congenital myasthenic syndrome. J Neurol 2013;260(3):815–9.
19. Hantai D, Richard P, Koenig J, et al. Congenital myasthenic syndromes. Curr Opin Neurol 2004;17(5):539–51.
20. Chaudhuri A, Behan PO. Myasthenic crisis. QJM 2009;102(2):97–107.
21. Riemersma S, Vincent A, Beeson D, et al. Association of arthrogryposis multiplex congenita with maternal antibodies inhibiting fetal acetylcholine receptor function. J Clin Invest 1996;98(10):2358–63.
22. American Academy of Pediatrics Committee on Drugs. Transfer of drugs and other chemicals into human milk. Pediatrics 2001;108(3):776–89.
23. Stickler DE, Stickler LL. Single-fiber electromyography during menstrual exacerbation and ovulatory suppression in MuSK antibody-positive myasthenia gravis. Muscle Nerve 2007;35(6):808–11.
24. How dangerous is the pill? Z Allgemeinmed 1975;(26):1156–7 [in German].

Connective Tissue Disorders in Pregnancy

Sophia L. Ryan, MD[a,b,c,*], Shamik Bhattacharyya, MD, MS[a,c]

KEYWORDS

- Connective tissue disorders • Systemic lupus erythematosus • Sjögren syndrome
- Idiopathic inflammatory myopathy • Marfan syndrome

KEY POINTS

- Both genetic and autoimmune causes of connective tissue disorders can affect women during childbearing years, and pregnancy is often associated with changes in disease activity.
- In patients with systemic lupus erythematosus, pregnancy is a period of increased disease flares, as well as an increased overall risk of mortality, thrombosis, infection, preterm labor, and preeclampsia.
- The course of Sjögren syndrome is thought to worsen during and after pregnancy with obstetric outcomes depending on maternal disease severity and antibody profile.
- In women affected by the inflammatory idiopathic myopathies, active disease during pregnancy appears to increase the risk of pregnancy loss, typically prompting treatment with steroids.
- Aortic root dissection is a life-threatening consequence of Marfan syndrome, the risk of which is increased during pregnancy.

INTRODUCTION

Connective tissue disorders broadly refer to diseases affecting the matrix that supports organ systems. As understanding of diseases has grown more specific, the term connective tissue disorders now encompasses 2 broad and pathogenically unrelated categories of disease. The first is genetic diseases, such as Marfan syndrome, Ehlers-Danlos syndrome, and fibromuscular dysplasia, with prominent abnormalities in skeletal and vascular tissue. The second is autoimmune diseases, such as systemic lupus erythematosus (SLE), Sjögren syndrome (SS), myositis, systemic sclerosis, and antiphospholipid syndrome. Both genetic and autoimmune causes of connective

Disclosure Statement: The authors do not have any relevant disclosures.
[a] Department of Neurology, Brigham and Women's Hospital, 75 Francis Street, Boston, MA 02115, USA; [b] Department of Neurology, Massachusetts General Hospital, 75 Francis Street, Boston, MA 02115, USA; [c] Department of Neurology, Harvard Medical School, 75 Francis Street, Boston, MA 02115, USA
* Corresponding author. 75 Francis Street, Boston, MA 02115.
E-mail address: sryan9@partners.org

tissue disorders can affect women during childbearing years, and pregnancy is often associated with changes in disease activity. Because of the many serious neurologic complications of these diseases, the neurologist is often consulted on management during pregnancy. We review here some of the more common diseases, their neurologic effects, and changes with pregnancy.

SYSTEMIC LUPUS ERYTHEMATOSUS

SLE is a systemic inflammatory disorder more common in women compared with men, becoming clinically manifest in most between the late teens and early 40s. SLE is a heterogeneous disease with variable clinical severity ranging from minor symptoms to refractory disease unresponsive to immunosuppression. The American College of Rheumatology formulated classification criteria in 1987 for SLE and required 4 of the following 11 features[1]:

1. Facial erythema over the malar eminences and/or bridge of the nose (malar rash)
2. Erythematous raised patches with keratotic scaling and follicular plugging (discoid lupus)
3. Photosensitivity defined as any skin reaction from exposure to sunlight
4. Oral or nasopharyngeal ulcers (often painless)
5. Nonerosive arthritis characterized by tenderness, swelling, or effusion of 2 or more peripheral joints
6. Serositis typically pleuritis or pericarditis
7. Renal disorder manifesting as proteinuria or cellular casts
8. Neurologic disorder broadly characterized by seizures or psychosis
9. Hematologic disorder consisting of hemolytic anemia, leukopenia, lymphopenia, or thrombocytopenia
10. Presence of antidouble-strand DNA (dsDNA), anti-Smith (Sm), or antiphospholipid antibodies
11. Presence of antinuclear antibody

These criteria were not developed to diagnose individual patients. Thus, patients may have SLE and not have 4 of the 11 features.

The pathogenesis of SLE is likely multifactorial, with contributions from genetic susceptibility, environmental factors, such as infection with Epstein-Barr virus, abnormalities in apoptosis, and hormonal factors.[2] SLE is associated with multiple autoantibodies frequently against intracellular components. The antinuclear antibody (ANA) is present in approximately 95% of patients, but the antibody is not specific and can be found in asymptomatic individuals or those with other autoimmune diseases. There have been more than 100 other autoantibodies described in SLE, although only a smaller subset is clinically tested. The anti-dsDNA antibody is less sensitive but correlates with disease activity. There are other antibodies, such as anti-Sm antibody, which are highly specific but insensitive.

SLE can injure both the central and peripheral nervous system. There have been a series of neuropathological studies published regarding the neurologic involvement of SLE. Most frequently, in the central nervous system, SLE is associated with injury to the small vessels causing microinfarcts from vasculopathy or in some cases from cardioembolism from Libman-Sacks endocarditis. Most importantly, although often invoked, "lupus vasculitis" is not a frequent cause of neurologic damage and rarely substantiated by pathology.[3] Other modes of injury include inflammation causing encephalitis. Although many have been proposed, there is not yet an autoantibody that is sufficiently sensitive or specific for neuropsychiatric lupus to be clinically useful. Some proposed examples include anti-ribosomal P antibody and anti-N-methyl-D-aspartate receptor NR2 subunit antibody. Historically, there have been many terms used to describe neurologic impairment in the setting of SLE, including neurolupus and lupus cerebritis. The current preferred term is neuropsychiatric SLE (NPSLE), which is agnostic of the mechanism of the injury (ie, not necessarily inflammatory as implied by lupus cerebritis). The estimated prevalence of neuropsychiatric involvement in SLE is approximately 56%, although the range varies.[4] The most frequent associated syndrome is headache followed by mood disorder, cognitive dysfunction, seizures, and cerebrovascular disease.

Systemically, pregnancy and the postpartum period are associated with increased risk of SLE flares. Among women with SLE, there is increased overall risk of mortality as well as of thrombosis, infection, preterm labor, and preeclampsia.[5] Generally, active disease before conception and history of lupus nephritis are associated with increased risk of SLE flare during pregnancy. There is scarcity of data on pregnancy outcomes in patients with NPSLE. There are many case reports describing individual patients with flares of NPSLE during pregnancy. The largest retrospective series describes 26 pregnancies in patients with current or prior history of NPSLE.[6] In this small series, there appeared to be an association with prematurity and preeclampsia consistent with what is known generally about SLE. Hence, how to manage neurologic syndromes during pregnancy is guided more by clinical experience than by data.

Even though headache is the most commonly associated neurologic complaint in SLE, headache in isolation is no more frequent in patients with SLE compared with the general population and does not correlate with SLE activity.[7] Neither tension type nor migraine headache is more prevalent in patients with SLE. Headache consequently is treated symptomatically during pregnancy. Importantly, headache in combination with other red flag symptoms, such as neck stiffness or postural headache, can indicate serious complications, such as aseptic meningitis or cerebral venous sinus thrombosis. Like headache, mood disorder is also frequent but the causality is less clear. Depression is commonly reported in SLE, and in controlled epidemiologic studies, elevated SLE disease activity increases the odds of major depression minimally, although contradictory results also have been reported.[8] On the other hand, psychosis is more closely related to disease activity and can be the presenting symptom of SLE. In patients with SLE and psychosis, an important secondary cause to exclude is steroid-induced psychosis. A clinical clue is that steroid-induced psychosis contains more prevalent auditory hallucinations whereas SLE psychosis has more prominent visual hallucinations. There is no clear biomarker for SLE-associated psychosis. The syndrome responds to immunosuppression.

Stroke is a major cause of morbidity and mortality in patients with SLE. In a 10-year prospective series of 1000 patients with SLE, stroke accounted for 12% of deaths and, as an individual cause of death, ranked second only behind infectious complications.[9] Overall, across all age groups, patients with SLE have a roughly twofold increased risk of stroke compared with the general population.[10] This increased risk is especially significant in the younger age groups in which the general population baseline risk is low. For example, in the 30 to 39 age group, there is a 21-fold increased risk of stroke in patients with SLE. The pathogenesis of stroke in the context of SLE is complex and likely involves multiple mechanisms, including accelerated small vessel disease in the arterioles, embolic infarcts both from infective and Libman-Sacks endocarditis, antiphospholipid syndrome, and accelerated large vessel atherosclerosis. Cerebral vasculitis is a rare and likely minor contributor to stroke in SLE. Of the various mechanisms, antiphospholipid syndrome is a major cause, and antiphospholipid antibodies are found in most patients with SLE who have an ischemic stroke. There are scarce data on changes in stroke risk with pregnancy in SLE and whether women who have experienced a stroke need to be treated differently. One important exception is antiphospholipid syndrome. Women with antiphospholipid antibody syndrome associated with ischemic stroke who become pregnant are generally treated with therapeutic low molecular weight heparin for the duration of the pregnancy.[11] Low-dose aspirin is often added to this regimen to reduce the risk of preeclampsia and because of higher risk of thrombotic recurrence with prior arterial thrombotic event.

Myelitis is relatively rare, with estimated prevalence of less than 1% and is likely of heterogeneous etiology. Some have longitudinally extensive myelitis and test positive for anti-Aquaporin 4 antibodies associated with the disease neuromyelitis optica (NMO). These patients also respond to treatment for NMO. Based on what is generally known about NMO, pregnancy is associated with increased relapse rate.[12] However, most patients will not test positive for NMO immunoglobulin G, and the pathophysiology remains unclear. Examination of cerebrospinal fluid (CSF) often shows inflammatory disease. Patients are generally treated with aggressive immunotherapy, including with cyclophosphamide, plasmapheresis, intravenous immunoglobulin, and rituximab. Some of these medications (such as cyclophosphamide) are contraindicated during pregnancy, and flares during pregnancy are generally treated with steroids.

Aside from these syndromes discussed, SLE has been associated with multiple neurologic syndromes, including cognitive impairment, different kinds of neuropathy, movement disorders, aseptic meningitis, posterior reversible encephalopathy syndrome, hypophysitis, and increased intracranial hypertension. During pregnancy, these disorders are treated individually rather than in an SLE-specific manner.

SJÖGREN SYNDROME

SS is a disease primarily of middle-aged women, affecting 2 to 4 million people in the United States. The average age of diagnosis is 55, but there is a bimodal distribution with peaks at ages 30 (during childbearing years) and 55 (just after menopause).[13] The female-to-male predominance is between 9 and 20:1, higher than for any other connective tissue disorder.[14] Clinically, for primary SS, 4 of the following 6 criteria are required: (1) ocular symptoms (typically for more than 3 months); (2) oral symptoms (typically for more than 3 months); (3) evidence of ocular exocrine dysfunction (ie, positive Schirmer test or Rose Bengal stain); (4) evidence of oral exocrine dysfunction (decreased whole salivary flow, abnormal parotid sialography, or abnormal salivary scintigraphy); (5) histopathology (salivary gland showing lymphocytic foci); or (6) serology positive for anti-Ro/SSA and/or anti-La/SSB. Other laboratory changes in SS include elevation of paraproteins, cryoglobulins, hypergammaglobulinemia and autoantibodies. Other commonly observed autoantibodies are ANAs and rheumatoid factor. Low complement (C3, C4) levels are also frequently observed in patients with SS. Some of these serologic changes are likely directly related to SS itself, whereas others are more likely due to other comorbid autoimmunity.

Pathologically, SS is characterized by lymphocytic infiltration of the exocrine glands: the salivary and lacrimal glands. Thus, SS frequently manifests as dry eyes and dry mouth, the so-called "sicca syndrome." In addition to the exocrine system, SS can involve many other organs, including the brain, lungs, kidneys, thyroid, muscle, and skin and give rise to a diverse set of extraglandular symptoms, including depression, pain, cutaneous lesions, and mild arthritis. The most common neurologic complaint, seen in 50% of patients with SS, is extreme fatigue.[15] It is more frequent in female than male patients, and is a major contributor to decreased functional status in patients with SS. SS is also associated with thyroid dysfunction, present in approximately 45% of patients, and more common in women than men. Subclinical hypothyroidism may be an important contributor to the fatigue seen in SS.[15]

Neurologically, SS affects both the central (CNS) and peripheral nervous system (PNS). Notably, neurologic manifestations frequently precede the onset of the more typical sicca symptoms, which can lead to a delay in diagnosis.[16] The PNS has traditionally been thought to be more commonly affected than the CNS, with 10% of patients diagnosed with peripheral neuropathy. Of these, predominantly sensory manifestations are most commonly reported. If one looks for subclinical changes in nerve conduction or intraepidermal nerve fiber density, estimates of peripheral nerve involvement in patients with SS increase to as high as 60%.[17] The range of neuropathies includes mixed polyneuropathy, axonal sensory neuropathy, sensory ataxic neuropathy, axon sensorimotor polyneuropathy, trigeminal or other cranial neuropathies, demyelinating polyradiculoneuropathy, autonomic neuropathy, pure sensory neuronopathy, mononeuritis multiplex, and small-fiber neuropathy. Raynaud phenomenon, which occurs in many connective tissue autoimmune diseases, including SS, is another symptom that may be a result of peripheral nerve dysfunction via dysregulation of autonomic and small nerve fibers resulting in prolonged vasoconstriction of peripheral vessels. This phenomenon may occur more frequently in women than men with SS.

The CNS is affected approximately between 2% and 60% of the time depending on how involvement is defined (with clear structural changes at the low end and functional changes including fatigue and headache at the higher end). In the CNS, SS can present similarly to multiple sclerosis with numerous white matter lesions, as a NMO spectrum disorder (with 90% of these patients showing seropositivity for Aquaporin-4 antibodies) or with recurrent aseptic meningoencephalitis (fever, headache, meningismus, confusion paired with CSF pleocytosis).[14] In addition to the more focal CNS manifestations, there is increasing evidence that SS can be accompanied by diffuse nonfocal neuropsychiatric manifestations. Depression and fibromyalgia, for example, are important CNS manifestations that affect women more commonly than men. Furthermore, on neuropsychiatric testing, patients often have frontal, executive. and verbal memory dysfunction. It remains unclear whether this is a direct effect of the disease, a psychological reaction to it, or a byproduct of treatment.

All treatment recommendations for the neurologic manifestations of SS are derived from small, retrospective case series. Possible disease-modifying drugs include IV immunoglobulin (IVIG), corticosteroids, plasmapheresis, rituximab, and infliximab. IVIG and corticosteroids have been shown in a small case series to bring about a 30% to 40% improvement in neuropathy.[18] This was further broken down by the type of peripheral neuropathy with multiple mononeuropathies seeming to respond best to corticosteroids, and painful neuropathy responding best to IVIG. Infliximab, rituximab, and plasmapheresis have also been used with anecdotal success. In addition to disease-modifying drugs, the neurologic symptoms resulting from SS can be treated with a variety of medications such as gabapentin, pregabalin, tricyclic antidepressants, duloxetine, and topical lidocaine, all of which are frequently used for neuropathic pain. As with most conditions, treatment of SS in women during pregnancy is fraught with concerns about potential teratogenicity butting up against the need to control symptoms and the potential harmful effects of active disease itself. Furthermore, cost and drug availability are at the forefront of any treatment decisions, particularly given that no standard of care exists in neurologic complications of SS due to the lack of randomized control trials.

There have been increasing pregnancies among women with SS in recent years. This is likely explained by the bimodal peaks of SS onset with 1 peak in the early 30s paired with trends toward women deferring pregnancy later. There has thus been increasing interest in the effect of SS on pregnancy and vice versa. Although data are still scarce, it appears that the course of SS is likely to worsen during and after pregnancy. This is thought to be related to pulmonary hypertension as a complication of SS.[19] Additionally, obstetric outcomes appear to be worse in women with SS, depending on the disease severity and antibody profile. Congenital heart block (CHB) as a manifestation of neonatal lupus is the best known and most severe complication observed in women with SS and is thought to be related to circulating maternal anti-Ro/SSA and anti-La/SSB antibodies. The occurrence rate of CHB is approximately 2% in infants born to women who are anti-Ro/SSA antibody positive and approximately 3% in infants born to women who are anti-La-SSB positive.[20] Outcomes in such infants with heart block are poor, with higher rates of morbidity and mortality, and most surviving infants requiring early permanent pacemaker placement. Maternal treatment with fluorinated steroids during pregnancy can reduce the antibody-mediated damage to nodal tissue. In addition to the known association with CHB, women with SS have increased rates of spontaneous abortions, preterm deliveries, lower neonatal birth weights, and increased frequency of cesarean deliveries. Some of these findings, however, appear to be confounded by advanced maternal age as compared with controls.

INFLAMMATORY IDIOPATHIC MYOPATHIES

The inflammatory idiopathic myopathies (IIMs) constitute an important, albeit rare, group of autoimmune diseases with neurologic involvement. IIMs involve immune-mediated attack of skeletal muscle resulting in weakness. Women are 3 times more likely to suffer from IIMs than men (excepting inclusion body myositis [IBM], which affects men 3 times more often than women). This, paired with the fact that an estimated 14% of patients with IIM develop disease before or during childbearing years, makes the issue of myositis in pregnancy of clinical importance to neurologists and obstetricians alike.

Although many classification systems for IIM exist, the most recent version proposed in 2017 by the European League Against Rheumatism/American College of Rheumatology has 5 subtypes: (1) dermatomyositis (DM), (2) polymyositis (PM), (3) amyopathic DM (ie, DM without muscle involvement), (4) juvenile DM, and (5) sporadic IBM.[21] Using these criteria paired with muscle biopsy, the sensitivity and specificity of a probable IIM diagnosis are 93% and 88%, respectively (87% and 82% without muscle biopsy). Electromyography and muscle MRI were excluded from the classification criteria (although certainly used clinically), and only a single myositis-specific antibody anti-Jo-1, was included. Other myopathies not included in this classification are cancer-associated myositis, overlap myositis (patients who also meet criteria for other autoimmune conditions), and necrotizing autoimmune myopathy.

Diagnosis of the IIMs remains challenging because of their clinical complexity, relative rarity, and overlapping characteristics. DM and PM are the most common IIMs. Both DM and PM are typically characterized by progressive symmetric proximal muscle weakness. The dermatologic distinguishing features of DM include heliotrope rash, Gottron papules, and Gottron sign. In DM, the key histopathological feature is perimysial inflammation, whereas in PM, muscle biopsy typically demonstrates endomysial inflammation. There is also an association between IIMs and malignancy. IBM is unique because of its more insidious onset over months and early involvement of distal finger flexors and quadriceps. DM and PM are typically treated initially with corticosteroids with addition of steroid-sparing therapy (such as azathioprine or mycophenolate) when prolonged therapy is necessary.[22] IBM is generally not responsive to immunosuppression.

IIMs can precede pregnancy (with or without disease flare during pregnancy), be present during pregnancy, shortly after pregnancy, or may appear after childbearing years. The literature around IIMs in pregnancy consists primarily of case reports or single-center cohort studies. In a series of 28 women with DM, PM, or an overlap syndrome, only 4 had IIM onset in proximity to pregnancy (5 total pregnancies), with the remainder experiencing disease onset after their childbearing years.[23] One of these pregnancies preceded disease onset by less than 1 year and was uneventful. The other 4 postdated disease onset. There were no documented cases of IIM diagnosis arising during pregnancy. Of those 4 pregnancies in women with preexisting disease, 2 suffered pregnancy loss, both of whom had active disease (1 a spontaneous abortion, albeit while on methotrexate, and 1 a late pregnancy loss). The other 2 were in remission at the time of pregnancy and had successful pregnancies. Based on similar series and compilation of other published cases, disease activity does not appear to increase during pregnancy (low-quality data). However, for those with active disease, there is likely a risk of pregnancy loss either as a consequence of the disease or possibly from the treatment. Hence, active inflammatory disease is typically treated with steroids, which is typically well tolerated during pregnancy.

GENETIC CONNECTIVE TISSUE DISORDERS

This group of diseases is heterogeneous and encompasses diseases with known causative mutations, such as Marfan syndrome (*fibrillin-1* mutation) and those without a single causative gene, such as fibromuscular dysplasia. The behavior of these diseases during pregnancy is individual for each disease. Some of these diseases, however, are associated with vasculopathies, of which Marfan syndrome (MFS) is a well characterized example. This multisystem disease is characterized most specifically by aortic root dilation and lens dislocation (ectopia lentis) in addition to a number of less specific features, including hypermobility, pectus abnormalities, dural ectasia, increased arm length to height ratio, pneumothorax, and scoliosis.[24] Of these manifestations, the most concerning one is aortic root dilation, which is often progressive with time. Left untreated, progressive aortic root dilation is associated with aortic dissection, which can be in the proximal (more common) or distal segments of the aorta and is a life-threatening emergency. Neurologically, proximal aortic root dissection and distal extension abruptly occlude the origins of the carotid or vertebral arteries and can result in large ischemic infarcts in the brain.

The risk of aortic root dissection is increased during pregnancy in MFS.[25] In fact, the most common cause of aortic dissection during pregnancy is MFS. The cause of this increased risk is unclear, but postulated mechanisms include changes in hemodynamics during pregnancy and hormonal effects on the vessel wall itself. The third trimester of pregnancy and early postpartum period are the times of highest risk for aortic root complications. Treatment of proximal aortic root dissection is emergent surgery to repair the dissection. When MFS is known before conception, active surveillance for aortic root dilation is recommended. The risk of dissection is dependent on the size of aortic root dilation, and prophylactic surgery is recommended on a consensus basis when the aortic root diameter is larger than 4.5 cm or shows rapid expansion.[24] In pregnant women with aortic root diameter smaller than 4.0 cm, medical management with beta-blockers is instituted.

FUTURE CONSIDERATIONS

Larger series will be critical to further characterize the behavior of these diseases in pregnancy, as well as their impact on mother and fetus alike. Further, as more and more therapeutics become available, their efficacy and safety in pregnancy will need to be better studied through both observational and experimental trials.

REFERENCES

1. Hochberg MC. Updating the American College of Rheumatology revised criteria for the classification of systemic lupus erythematosus. Arthritis Rheum 1997; 40(9):1725.
2. D'Cruz DP, Khamashta MA, Hughes GRV. Systemic lupus erythematosus. Lancet 2007;369(9561):587–96.
3. Johnson RT, Richardson EP. The neurological manifestations of systemic lupus erythematosus. Medicine (Baltimore) 1968;47(4):337–69.
4. Unterman A, Nolte JES, Boaz M, et al. Neuropsychiatric syndromes in systemic lupus erythematosus: a meta-analysis. Semin Arthritis Rheum 2011;41(1):1–11.
5. Clowse MEB, Jamison M, Myers E, et al. A national study of the complications of lupus in pregnancy. Am J Obstet Gynecol 2008;199(2):127.e1–6.
6. de Jesus GR, Rodrigues BC, Lacerda MI, et al. Gestational outcomes in patients with neuropsychiatric systemic lupus erythematosus. Lupus 2017;26(5):537–42.
7. Mitsikostas DD, Sfikakis PP, Goadsby PJ. A meta-analysis for headache in systemic lupus erythematosus: the evidence and the myth. Brain 2004;127(Pt 5): 1200–9.
8. Palagini L, Mosca M, Tani C, et al. Depression and systemic lupus erythematosus: a systematic review. Lupus 2013;22(5):409–16.
9. Cervera R, Khamashta MA, Font J, et al. Morbidity and mortality in systemic lupus erythematosus during a 10-year period: a comparison of early and late manifestations in a cohort of 1,000 patients. Medicine (Baltimore) 2003;82(5):299–308. Available at: https://www.ncbi.nlm.nih.gov/pubmed/14530779. Accessed February 19, 2018.
10. Schoenfeld SR, Kasturi S, Costenbader KH. The epidemiology of atherosclerotic cardiovascular disease among patients with SLE: a systematic review. Semin Arthritis Rheum 2013;43(1):77–95.
11. Bates SM, Greer IA, Middeldorp S, et al. VTE, thrombophilia, antithrombotic therapy, and pregnancy: antithrombotic therapy and prevention of thrombosis, 9th edition: American College of Chest Physicians evidence-based clinical practice guidelines. Chest 2012;141(2 Suppl):e691S–736S.
12. Davoudi V, Keyhanian K, Bove RM, et al. Immunology of neuromyelitis optica during pregnancy. Neurol Neuroimmunol Neuroinflamm 2016;3(6):e288.
13. Brandt JE, Priori R, Valesini G, et al. Sex differences in Sjögren's syndrome: a comprehensive review of immune mechanisms. Biol Sex Differ 2015;6:19.
14. Bhattacharyya S, Helfgott SM. Neurologic complications of systemic lupus erythematosus, Sjögren syndrome, and rheumatoid arthritis. Semin Neurol 2014; 34(4):425–36.
15. Kassan SS, Moutsopoulos HM. Clinical manifestations and early diagnosis of Sjögren syndrome. Arch Intern Med 2004;164(12):1275–84.
16. Delalande S, de Seze J, Fauchais A-L, et al. Neurologic manifestations in primary Sjögren syndrome: a study of 82 patients. Medicine (Baltimore) 2004;83(5): 280–91.

17. Chai J, Logigian EL. Neurological manifestations of primary Sjogren's syndrome. Curr Opin Neurol 2010;23(5):509–13.
18. Mori K, Iijima M, Koike H, et al. The wide spectrum of clinical manifestations in Sjögren's syndrome-associated neuropathy. Brain 2005;128(Pt 11):2518–34.
19. Gupta S, Gupta N. Sjögren syndrome and pregnancy: a literature review. Perm J 2017;21 [pii:16-047].
20. De Carolis S, Salvi S, Botta A, et al. The impact of primary Sjogren's syndrome on pregnancy outcome: our series and review of the literature. Autoimmun Rev 2014; 13(2):103–7.
21. Bottai M, Tjärnlund A, Santoni G, et al. EULAR/ACR classification criteria for adult and juvenile idiopathic inflammatory myopathies and their major subgroups: a methodology report. RMD Open 2017;3(2):e000507.
22. Dalakas MC. Inflammatory muscle diseases. N Engl J Med 2015;372(18): 1734–47.
23. Silva CA, Sultan SM, Isenberg DA. Pregnancy outcome in adult-onset idiopathic inflammatory myopathy. Rheumatology (Oxford) 2003;42(10):1168–72.
24. Loeys BL, Dietz HC, Braverman AC, et al. The revised Ghent nosology for the Marfan syndrome. J Med Genet 2010;47(7):476–85.
25. Goland S, Elkayam U. Pregnancy and Marfan syndrome. Ann Cardiothorac Surg 2017;6(6):642–53.

Stroke in Pregnancy
An Update

Erica C. Camargo, MD, MMSc, PhD[a], Steven K. Feske, MD[b],
Aneesh B. Singhal, MD[c],*

KEYWORDS

- Ischemic stroke • Hemorrhagic stroke • Pregnancy
- Hypertensive disorders of pregnancy

KEY POINTS

- Pregnancy and puerperium confer a substantially increased risk of ischemic and hemorrhagic stroke in women, the rates of which have increased approximately 50% to 80% over the past 20 years.
- The period of highest risk of stroke is the peripartum/postpartum phase, coinciding with the highest risk for hypertensive disorders of pregnancy and peak risk of gestational hypercoagulability.
- Hemorrhagic stroke is the most common type of obstetric stroke, most commonly associated with hypertensive disorders of pregnancy.
- Hypertensive disorders of pregnancy are among the most important contributors to obstetric stroke and may predispose women to premature cardiovascular disease later in life.
- Other conditions associated with stroke in pregnancy include posterior reversible encephalopathy, reversible cerebral vasoconstriction syndrome, and cerebral venous sinus thrombosis.

EPIDEMIOLOGY
Incidence, Prevalence, and Temporal Trends

Pregnancy and puerperium confer an increased risk for ischemic as well as hemorrhagic stroke, with incidence rates being 3-fold higher as compared with nonpregnant women. A recent meta-analysis of the epidemiologic characteristics and risk factors for stroke in pregnancy found that the mean age ranged from 22 to 33 years, and the crude incidence rate was 30/100,000 (95% confidence interval [CI],

Disclosures: None.
[a] Department of Neurology, Massachusetts General Hospital, Harvard Medical School, 55 Fruit Street, Boston, MA 02114, USA; [b] Stroke Division, Department of Neurology, Brigham and Women's Hospital, Harvard Medical School, 25 Shattuck Street, Boston, MA 02115, USA; [c] Department of Neurology, Massachusetts General Hospital, Harvard Medical School, 55 Fruit Street, WACC 729-C, Boston, MA 02114, USA
* Corresponding author.
E-mail address: asinghal@partners.org

Neurol Clin 37 (2019) 131–148
https://doi.org/10.1016/j.ncl.2018.09.010
0733-8619/19/© 2018 Elsevier Inc. All rights reserved.

neurologic.theclinics.com

18.8–49.4/100,000).[1] The rate of ischemic and hemorrhagic stroke was 12.2/100,000 pregnancies, whereas for cerebral venous sinus thrombosis (CVST) the rate was 9.1/100,000 pregnancies. In this meta-analysis, the rates of pregnancy-associated stroke remained unchanged from 1990 to 2017.[1] However, using hospital discharge data from the US Nationwide Inpatient Sample, Kuklina and colleagues[2] reported that the rate of stroke from 1994 to 1995 to 2006 to 2007 increased by 47% for antenatal stroke and by 83% for postnatal strokes. Changes in the prevalence of hypertensive disorders of pregnancy (HDP) and heart disease from 1994 to 1995 to 2006 to 2007 explained almost all the increase in postpartum hospitalizations. Such changes in the incidence of stroke have not yet been replicated in other studies[2]; better stroke detection and reporting may partly explain this increase.

Timing

The rate of prepartum/peripartum stroke is 18.3/100,000 pregnancies, whereas for postpartum stroke the rate is 14.7/100,000. Given the short duration of the postpartum period, the daily rate of stroke is higher in the postpartum as compared with pre- or peripartum periods.[1] Different rates have been reported in England: 10.7/100,000 person-years, antepartum, but 9-fold higher peripartum (161.1/100,000 person-years) and 3-fold higher early postpartum (47.1/100,000 person-years).[3] It is postulated that these differences could be due to variances in access to obstetric care between the United States and England. The postpartum period with highest risk for thrombotic events is the first 6 weeks. Although the period of 7 to 12 weeks postpartum also has an increased, albeit lower, risk of thrombotic events compared with weeks 0 to 6, there is no significant increase in stroke risk.[4]

RISK FACTORS
Patient Characteristics

A study of the Nationwide Inpatient Sample showed that the absolute risk of stroke increased with age: compared with patients younger than 20 years, those aged 35 to 39 years had an odds ratio (OR) for stroke of 2.0 (95% CI 1.4–2.7, $P<.01$) and those older than or equal to 40 years had OR of 3.1 (95% CI 2–4.6).[5] One study found that younger women, but not older women, had an increased stroke risk during pregnancy and the postpartum state.[6] Pregnancy at older age may, however, have negative implications for cerebrovascular health later in life. The risk of stroke in relation to age of prior pregnancy/delivery was analyzed in women aged 59 to 70 years from the observational cohort of the Women's Health Study. Older age at delivery (age ≥40 years) was associated with a small but significant increased risk of hemorrhagic stroke in multivariate analyses (OR 1.5, 95% CI 1.0–2.1) compared with women younger than 40 years at delivery. Compared with younger women at the time of delivery, women older than or equal to 40 years at delivery had higher mean systolic blood pressure and higher rates of diabetes mellitus, heart failure, atrial fibrillation, and any alcohol use later in life.[7]

Data from the Nationwide Inpatient Sample also showed that Race/Ethnicity influences the incidence of pregnancy-associated stroke: African-American women have higher risk of stroke than White women (OR 1.5, 95% CI 1.2–1.9) and Hispanic women.[5]

Medical Risk Factors

The presence of vascular risk factors at the time of pregnancy contributes to the risk of stroke. Medical conditions that are strongly associated with stroke include the following: migraine, OR 16.9 (95% CI 9.7–29.5); thrombophilia, OR 16.0 (95% CI 9.4–27.2); systemic lupus erythematosus, OR 15.2 (95% CI 7.4–31.2); heart disease, OR 13.2 (95% CI 10.2–17.0); sickle cell disease, OR 9.1 (95% CI 3.7–22.2); hypertension, OR 6.1 (95% CI 4.5–8.1); thrombocytopenia, OR 6.0 (95% CI 1.5–24.1); and diabetes, OR 2.5 (95% CI 1.3–4.6). In addition, pregnancy-associated complications such as transfusion, postpartum infections, and any type of infection at the time of delivery admission, especially genitourinary infections and sepsis, are strong predictors of pregnancy-associated stroke.[5,8] Furthermore, smoking is highly prevalent in women who suffer strokes during pregnancy.[9] Other pregnancy-specific causes, such as peripartum cardiomyopathy, choriocarcinoma, and embolization of amniotic fluid or air, are very rare.

For hemorrhagic stroke during pregnancy/puerperium, aneurysms, arteriovenous malformations, and HDP are the most important risk factors.[1]

Assisted Reproductive Therapies

Conflicting data have been reported regarding the risk of cardiovascular disease and stroke after hormonally assisted reproductive therapies. A recent meta-analysis involving 30,477 women who received fertility therapy and 1,296,734 women who did not, who were respectively followed for a median of 9.7 and 8.6 years, showed a trend toward an increased risk of stroke or transient ischemic attack in women after ovulation induction compared with women who did not receive fertility therapy (hazard ratio, 1.25, 95% CI 0.96–1.63; $I^2$0%). It is noteworthy that the patients included in the studies were relatively young, with mean age of 28.5 to 34 years at the time of delivery, which could have biased the results toward a more favorable outcome.[10]

A prospective cohort study analyzed the risk of cardiovascular disease after failed assisted reproductive therapy (defined as women who did not give birth 1 year after their last cycle of assisted reproductive therapy) in 28,442 women who received fertility therapy, after a median of 8.4 years of follow-up. A total of 67% failed reproductive therapy and had a 21% increased annual risk of cardiovascular disease (95% CI 13%–30%) and an increased risk of ischemic stroke (adjusted relative rate ratio (ARR) 1.33, 95% CI 1.22 to 1.46) but not hemorrhagic stroke (ARR 0.88, 95% CI 0.80–0.96).[11]

The mechanisms by which assisted reproduction increases the risk of cardiovascular disease are not fully understood. It is postulated that ovarian hyperstimulation activates the renin-angiotensin system, thus modifying sodium balance, blood pressure regulation, and promoting fluid shifts with intravascular volume depletion, leading to hypercoagulability.

Cesarean Delivery

In a study of data from the Healthcare Cost and Utilization Project from 1993 and 1994, risk factors for peripartum stroke and venous sinus thrombosis were assessed among 1,408,015 sampled deliveries. In that study, the risk of peripartum stroke was 34.3/100,000 births for women who had a cesarean birth compared with risk of 7.1/100,000 births for vaginal delivery ($P<.001$). The risk of intracranial venous thrombosis was also increased for cesarean delivery: 26.6/100,000 births for cesarean birth versus 7.4/100,000 births for vaginal delivery ($P<.001$).[12] Similar findings were observed in a population-based study from Taiwan, in which the increased risk of postpartum stroke in women undergoing cesarean delivery compared with vaginal delivery persisted up to 12 months postpartum.[13] The possibility of cesarean section being a consequence of pregnancies complicated by HDP, for which the risk of stroke is higher due to hypertension or due to the actual occurrence of a cerebrovascular event, is a potential confounder. However, surgery itself promotes increased risk of clotting through various mechanisms, which may account for the increased stroke risk.[12]

PATHOPHYSIOLOGY OF PREGNANCY-ASSOCIATED STROKE
Hemodynamic Changes

During pregnancy, there is a high metabolic demand. To account for this, cardiovascular changes occur to allow the maternal circulation to meet new physiologic requirements. One of the initial changes is an increase in the plasmatic volume beginning early in the first trimester, secondary to an increase in renin activity as stimulated by estrogen and other circulating hormones. There is also development of mild hemodilutional anemia, and substantial increases in heart rate and cardiac output, with elevation up to 45% more than the nonpregnancy state by 24 weeks, and even further during labor and birth.[14,15]

Systemic vascular resistance drops in early gestation. With this, blood pressure (BP) drops as well, with nadir around 20 to 32 weeks. This promotes relative venous stasis, heightened by vena cava compression in the supine position by the progressively growing uterus and reduced physical activity during late pregnancy and puerperium. Therefore, the combination of hypervolemia, increased circulatory demand, decreased BP, and increased venous stasis predispose women to circulatory complications. These changes persist until 6 to 12 weeks postpartum.

Vascular and Connective Tissue Changes

Pregnancy causes remodeling of the heart and blood vessels, with increased vascular distensibility in the first trimester. In late pregnancy, however, there is loss of distensibility due to a reduction in collagen and elastin content in the systemic arterial walls, which persists for months after delivery.[16] It is not clear how these vascular changes promote the development of stroke. However, it is postulated that these somewhat vulnerable vessel walls could be subject to greater hemodynamic stress in the setting of increased blood volume and cardiac output during pregnancy and delivery and hence susceptible to rupture and resultant hemorrhagic stroke.[9,15]

Changes in the Coagulation System

Gestation is a hypercoagulable state, with a 4- to 10-fold increased risk of thrombosis during pregnancy and puerperium. The increased hypercoagulability is in part due to elevations of procoagulant factors VII, IX, X, XII, and XIII; fibrinogen; and von Willebrand factor. Further, physiologic anticoagulation is partly impaired by reductions in protein S activity, reductions of antithrombin III levels (nadir in the third trimester), and development of acquired activated protein C resistance in the second and third trimesters in one-third of pregnant women. Fibrinolysis is also reduced because of increases in serum plasminogen activator inhibitor (PAI) type 1 and placental-derived PAI type 2. Iron deficiency also contributes to a procoagulant state. All these changes, combined with venous stasis, congestion, and compression of the inferior vena cava and aorta by the pregnant uterus promote an enhanced hypercoagulable state predominantly in the third trimester and puerperium. Further contributing to the risk of thrombosis in the puerperium is the acute phase response to surgical trauma and hemorrhage of delivery.[9,15,17]

PATHOLOGIC CONDITIONS, CONDITION-SPECIFIC MANAGEMENT, AND OUTCOMES
Hypertensive Disorders of Pregnancy

HDP are a group of conditions occurring in pregnancy and puerperium with a common background of hypertension, defined as BP greater than or equal to 140/90 mm Hg. Included in this group are gestational hypertension, preeclampsia, severe preeclampsia (eclampsia and hemolysis, elevated liver enzymes, and low platelets syndrome), and chronic hypertension with superimposed preeclampsia. HDP are of clinical relevance, given their prevalence and strong risk of cardiovascular disease and stroke during pregnancy and the puerperium and later in life, with associated increased risk of cardiovascular mortality.[18–20] Preeclampsia is associated with a 4-fold increase in future incident heart failure and a 2-fold increased risk in coronary heart disease, stroke, and death.[20] HDP lead to loss of women's premenopausal cardiovascular advantage, and cardiovascular disease may occur a decade earlier than expected.

The prevalence of HDP, gestational hypertension, and preeclampsia is 5.2% to 8.2%, 1.8% to 4.4%, and 0.2% to 9.2%, respectively. HDP is more common in developing countries, although its prevalence has increased substantially in the United States in the past 20 years.[21,22] HDP is also more common in African-Americans.[21]

Modifiable risk factors for HDP include increased body mass index, anemia, and lower education. Nonmodifiable risk factors for HDP include older and younger age (age >35 years and <20 years, respectively); primiparity and multiparity; previous HDP; gestational diabetes mellitus; preexisting hypertension; preexisting type 2 diabetes mellitus; preexisting urinary tract infection; and a family history of hypertension, type 2 diabetes mellitus, and preeclampsia.[21] In addition, coagulopathies, and underlying prothrombotic conditions also increase the risk of pregnancy-associated stroke in women with preeclampsia.[23]

HDP are associated with 26% of maternal deaths in Latin America/Caribbean and 16% of maternal deaths in developing countries. HDP also account for 10% of preterm births and 1/50 stillbirths.[24]

HDP are associated with a 1.7- to 5.2-fold increase in the risk of stroke. Furthermore, preeclampsia occurs in 21% to 47% of pregnancy-associated strokes.[5,25] Importantly, the rate of stroke associated with HDP increased 103% in the United States between the periods 1994 to 1995 and 2010 to 2011.[26]

Hypertension in pregnancy may predate the gestation or may be diagnosed de novo during pregnancy.

de novo hypertension

1. Gestational hypertension: diagnosed when hypertension develops in a woman at more than or equal to 20 weeks' gestation, in the absence of proteinuria or other metabolic abnormalities.[27] It may be mild, when BP ranges from 140 to 149/90 to 99 mm Hg; moderate when BP is 150 to 159/100 to 109 mm Hg; and severe when BP is greater than or equal to 160/110 mm Hg. Gestational hypertension is usually a relatively benign condition. However, 25% of women with gestational hypertension may develop preeclampsia, and those that have gestational hypertension before 34 weeks' gestation are at highest risk.

2. Preeclampsia: a multisystem disorder of mid- to late pregnancy diagnosed by the presence of de novo hypertension after 20 weeks' gestation accompanied by proteinuria (≥300 mg protein/24 hours urine) or evidence of maternal acute kidney injury, liver dysfunction, neurologic changes (encephalopathy, seizures), hemolysis or thrombocytopenia, or fetal growth restriction. Preeclampsia may occur

intrapartum and less frequently early postpartum, usually within 48 hours. Eclampsia, one of the most dreaded consequences of preeclampsia, is the development of seizures in a patient with preeclampsia. This occurs in about 0.1% of all pregnancies and is 10 to 30 times more common in developing countries.[21,28]

The pathophysiology of preeclampsia is not fully understood. There is evidence that immune maladaptation is central to its cause. Abnormal placentation, leading to restricted placental blood flow, may be the key factor promoting a cascade of events culminating with preeclampsia. Restricted placental blood flow leads to development of a necrotizing spiral artery arteriopathy, coined acute atherosis, which resembles the early stages of systemic atherosclerosis. The resultant placental oxidative and endoplasmic reticulum stress leads to the release of components from the intervillous space into the maternal circulation, promoting maternal intravascular inflammatory response (increase in tumor necrosis factor alpha, interleukin 6 (IL-6), intercellular adhesion molecule 1, C-reactive protein, and IL-2), generalized endothelial dysfunction, immune and clotting activation, decreased intravascular volume, and increased vascular reactivity. Microthrombi may be seen in multiple organs.[24,29]

The importance of diagnosis and early management of preeclampsia cannot be overstated. The maternal mortality rate in preeclampsia-eclampsia is 6.4/10,000 cases at delivery, with nearly 20-fold increased risk of maternal mortality when preeclampsia develops before 32 weeks' gestation.[30] The most common type of stroke occurring after preeclampsia is hemorrhagic stroke, usually present in the postpartum period.[25] In addition, there is a clear overlap syndrome of postpartum angiopathy or the reversible cerebral vasoconstriction syndrome (RCVS), posterior reversible encephalopathy syndrome (PRES), and preeclampsia/eclampsia.[28] The relative risk of stroke occurring later in life after preeclampsia is 1.76 (95% CI, 1.40–2.22) for nonfatal stroke and RR = 2.98 (95% CI, 1.11–7.96) for fatal stroke.[31]

Management

1. Aspirin: aspirin was first shown to reduce the risk of preeclampsia in women in 1979.[32] Thereafter, it has been studied in multiple clinical trials. A recent study showed that for patients at high risk of developing preeclampsia, aspirin, 150 mg daily, from weeks 11 to 14 to week 36 of gestation, was superior to placebo for prevention of preterm preeclampsia (1.6% vs 4.3%, respectively, OR 0.38, 95% CI 0.20–0.74), without increasing the risk of poor neonatal outcomes.[33] This therapy has been recommended in the recently published consensus statement on hypertensive disorders of pregnancy from the International Society for the Study of Hypertension in Pregnancy (ISSHP).[27]
2. Calcium: high calcium intake during pregnancy has been shown to be associated with a reduced incidence of preeclampsia. The mechanism whereby calcium might mediate this effect is through reduction of parathyroid hormone release and reduction of intracellular calcium, leading to decreased smooth muscle contractility. In addition, calcium supplementation could also reduce uterine smooth muscle contractility and prevent preterm labor and delivery.[34–36] Calcium supplementation, 1.2 to 2.5 g/d is also recommended, in addition to aspirin, for women at high risk of preeclampsia who have low daily calcium intake or in whom the daily intake of calcium cannot be estimated.[27]
3. Hypertension management: for patients with severe hypertension (BP $\geq$160/110) during pregnancy/puerperium, BP should be controlled in a monitored setting, with agents including intravenous labetalol or hydralazine or oral nifedipine.

Management recommendations of moderate hypertension vary by medical society. For example, the American College of Obstetricians and Gynecologists does not recommend treatment of mild or moderate hypertension.[37] Conversely, a 2014 statement from the American Heart Association (AHA) suggests consideration of treatment of moderate hypertension in pregnancy.[38] The divergent opinions stem from concerns regarding (1) fetal outcomes, because aggressive BP control may lead to low birth weight due to relative placental insufficiency and (2) maternal outcomes, given increased maternal stroke risk and risk of development of severe hypertension during gestation. A 2015 randomized controlled clinical trial addressed this question. In that study, 987 pregnant women at 14 to 33 weeks' gestation, with nonproteinuric hypertension or gestational hypertension, were randomized to BP control with target diastolic BP 100 mm Hg (control group) or target diastolic BP 85 mm Hg. The primary outcome (pregnancy loss or high-level neonatal care >48 hours in the first 28 postnatal days) occurred in 31.4% of controls and in 30.7% receiving aggressive BP control (adjusted OR 1.02, 95% CI 0.77–1.35). There was also no significant difference in the percentage of infants with low birth weight between the 2 groups. Serious maternal complications did not differ between the study arms.[39] Since the reporting of this study's results, the ISSHP has recommended treatment of any type of maternal hypertension, aiming for target diastolic BP of 85 mm Hg.[27]

4. Magnesium sulfate: this is recommended for women with preeclampsia who have proteinuria and severe hypertension, or hypertension with neurologic signs or symptoms.[27] The use of magnesium sulfate in preeclamptic women with severe features has been shown to reduce the rate of progression to eclampsia by 58%, as compared with placebo.[40] Magnesium sulfate is also superior to diazepam and phenytoin for prevention of recurrent seizures in eclampsia.[41,42]

5. Regular exercise during pregnancy to maintain appropriate body weight is recommended, because that will reduce the likelihood of hypertension.[27]

Posterior Reversible Encephalopathy

Posterior reversible encephalopathy (PRES) refers to a syndrome of hypertensive encephalopathy characterized by reversible brain edema. This usually occurs in the setting of elevated BP or relative hypertension (compared with a patient's baseline BP). Patients typically present with headache, visual symptoms referable to the occipital lobes, and seizures. The disease may be complicated by cerebral hemorrhages and ischemic strokes.

There is an overlap between PRES and severe preeclampsia/eclampsia.[43] A small single-center retrospective cohort study showed radiological features that suggest PRES in 98% of women with eclampsia.[44] Similarly, another small retrospective cohort study reported radiological features that suggest PRES in 92% of women with eclampsia and in 19% of women with preeclampsia.[45]

The typical radiographic appearance of PRES is that of subcortical white matter and cortical edema in the bilateral parietal and occipital lobes. In less typical PRES, there can be extension to the frontal lobes, inferior temporal lobes, cerebellar hemispheres, brainstem, and deep white matter.[46] MR diffusion-weighted imaging can also show restricted diffusion and intracranial hemorrhages. Atypical radiological features and intracranial hemorrhages are less commonly seen in obstetric PRES.[47]

The goals of therapy are to normalize systemic BP, control seizures, and minimize vasospasm and risk of secondary infarct and hemorrhage.

Outcomes in nonobstetrical PRES may be more severe than that of patients with obstetric PRES, which may be driven by the severity of the underlying comorbidities in that population.[48]

Reversible Cerebral Vasoconstriction Syndrome

RCVS denotes a group of diseases characterized by segmental narrowing and dilatation of multiple intracranial arteries of days to weeks' duration.[49–52] RCVS is relatively rare, with a woman to man ratio of 2:10 to 10:1, and mean age of 42 to 44 years.[51,53,54] The most common presenting sign is recurrent thunderclap headache over days to weeks, sometimes progressing to persistent moderate headache. Focal neurologic deficits, such as hemiparesis, aphasia, and altered mental status, occur in 8% to 43%.[51,53,55] Visual changes are common, including blurriness, cortical visual loss, and Balint syndrome.[53] Generalized tonic-clonic seizures occur in 1% to 17% at disease onset.

The pathophysiology is uncertain. RCVS may occur due to spontaneous or provoked failed regulation of cerebral vascular tone, likely related to serotoninergic pathways and sympathetic overactivity.[50,57] RCVS has been associated with exposure to vasoactive drugs (antidepressants, nasal decongestants, triptans, cannabis, nicotine patches, cocaine, methamphetamine, amphetamine, lysergic acid), catecholamine-secreting tumors, immunosuppressants, blood products, uncontrolled hypertension, head trauma, and sexual activity. This condition has been seen in the postpartum state, with or without preeclampsia/eclampsia.[50,51,53,56–64] There may be overlapping mechanisms between RCVS and posterior reversible leukoencephalopathy syndrome (PRES), given the presence of reversible cerebral edema in 8% to 38% of RCVS cases, angiographic changes in patients with PRES, and similar clinical presentation between the 2 conditions (**Fig. 1**).[51,53,57,65,66]

Brain parenchymal imaging is often normal on admission, but changes may be seen over time in 81%, including ischemic strokes, intraparenchymal hemorrhages (42%), and convexal nonaneurysmal subarachnoid hemorrhages.[51,53,54,65,67] Vasogenic edema that suggests PRES is seen in 28%. Vascular imaging (computed tomographic [CT] angiography, MR angiography, or conventional transfemoral angiography) demonstrates multifocal areas of smooth arterial tapering and alternating dilatation. Initial angiographic studies may be normal in RCVS. Angiographic findings typically resolve within 90 days.[54]

RCVS and PRES may co-occur: radiological feature of PRES has been reported in 9% of patients with RCVS.[68] In addition, cases have been reported of women with clinico-radiological features of RCVS overlapping with PRES. In such cases, imaging shows posterior white and often gray matter change consistent with vasogenic cerebral edema or segmental narrowing and dilation of large- and medium-sized cerebral arteries, the findings typical of RCVS.[57]

RCVS is best managed conservatively, with discontinuation of the offending agent, symptomatic treatment for headache and agitation, bed rest and stool softeners to avoid the Valsalva maneuver, and avoidance of physical exertion. Antiplatelets are not recommended. BP should be allowed to autorregulate and BP drops avoided. Calcium channel blockers can be used for headache relief although they are often administered to treat the "vasospasm." Logically, patients should avoid exposure to precipitants of the disease as far as possible; however there is no evidence that reexposure precipitates RCVS.[50,56]

The outcome in RCVS is favorable, with more than 90% of patients having no disability. However, less than 5% have an aggressive course, with progression of vasospasm, severe neurologic disability, or death. This might be more common in postpartum RCVS.[62,69,70]

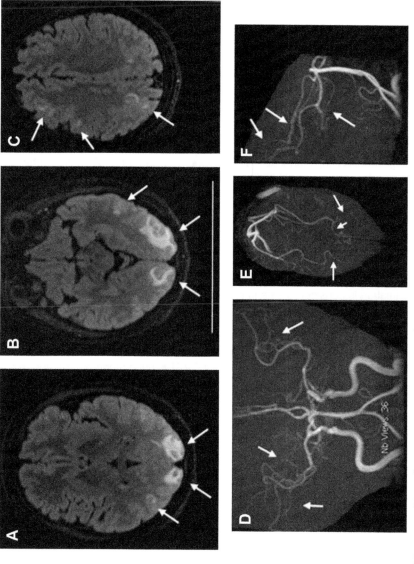

Fig. 1. 28-year-old woman, 34 weeks' gestation, presenting with 2-week history of unwell feeling and a 3-day history of nausea and headaches, followed by a generalized tonic-clonic seizure. Her admission blood pressure was 190/110. The patient was diagnosed with eclampsia and treated with

Cerebral Venous Sinus Thrombosis

CVST is an uncommon cerebrovascular disease characterized by thrombosis of the dural sinuses and cerebral veins, with resultant venous congestion, focal cerebral edema, and ultimately hemorrhagic venous infarctions. CVST accounts for 0.5% to 1% of all strokes.[71] CVST is most commonly seen in patients younger than 50 years, and 75% are women.[72] The most common risk factor is oral contraceptive use (54%). Genetic and acquired thrombophilias are seen in 34%. Other conditions include malignancy, hematologic disorders, pregnancy in 6.3%, puerperium in 13.8%, and infections. Forty-four percent of patients may have a combination of risk factors.[72] Obstetric CVST is most commonly associated with hypertension, cesarean delivery, and infection.[12]

The most common presenting symptoms include headache (88%),[73–75] seizures (40%), papilledema (30%), visual loss, diplopia, fluctuating motor or sensory deficits, stupor, and coma.[72] The disease affects most commonly the superior sagittal sinus (62%), the transverse sinus (41%–45%), straight sinus (18%), cortical veins (17%), and deep venous system (11%).[72]

The diagnosis of CVST requires high degree of clinical suspicion. Cerebral venous imaging is required for diagnosis, preferably performed with CT venography and MR venography. MR susceptibility-weighted imaging is useful for the diagnosis of CVST, especially for cortical vein thrombosis.[76] Indirect parenchymal signs may be seen in CVST, which are most conspicuous on brain MRI. These vary from normal appearing parenchyma to focal edema, cerebral hemorrhages, and increased or decreased water diffusivity (**Fig. 2**).[77]

The mainstay of treatment of CVST is clot dissolution with anticoagulation. In the acute phase, unfractionated heparin or low-molecular-weight heparin (LMWH) are recommended, followed by anticoagulation with warfarin for at least 3 to 6 months. Anticoagulation is considered safe in the presence of intracranial hemorrhage. However, in the peripartum period this may be complicated by risk of bleeding postdelivery or cesarean surgery. The duration of anticoagulation depends on the underlying condition. Thrombectomy is not routinely performed in CVST.

CVST is usually a benign condition, whereby 87% of patients will have none to mild deficits. Death occurs in 8.3%.[72,78] Recurrent CVST is uncommon (2.2%), and recurrent venous thromboembolic disease in recurrent pregnancies is infrequent.[79] Seizures can occur in 10.6% of patients. Any venous thromboembolic event can occur in 5.8% of patients, especially in the first year. Severe headaches can unfortunately persist after CVST in 14% of cases.[72]

Hemorrhagic Stroke

Pregnancy increases the risk for hemorrhagic much more than for ischemic stroke, with relative risk 2.5 during pregnancy and 28.5 postpartum.[80] Hemorrhagic stroke is an important cause of pregnancy-related mortality. The major established causes

---

labetalol, magnesium, and urgent induction of delivery. Brain MR axial FLAIR images (*A–C*) show hyperintense signal predominantly involving the subcortical white matter, but also extending to a lesser extent to the cortex, within (*A*) the bilateral occipital lobes, (*A*) right superior parietal lobe, (*B*) left middle temporal gyrus, and (*C*) right middle frontal gyrus and precentral gyrus. Magnetic resonance angiography of the brain (*D–F*) shows minimal luminal irregularity within (*D*) the middle cerebral arteries predominantly distally, as well as multifocal areas of mild narrowing within (*E, F*) the distal posterior cerebral arteries. These imaging findings suggest the PRES/RCVS overlap syndrome seen in preeclampsia/eclampsia.

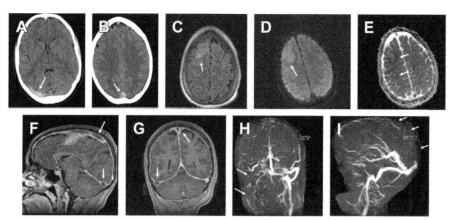

Fig. 2. A 29-year-old woman developed a headache 2 days after cesarean delivery, which progressed in intensity over 10 days, culminating with left-sided weakness and a seizure. Neuroimaging disclosed extensive venous sinus thrombosis involving the superior sagittal sinus, right lateral sinus, and right internal jugular vein, and a non-hemorrhagic venous infarction. Axial non-contrast head CT shows hyperdense thrombus (*arrows*) in the right transverse sinus (*A*) and superior sagittal sinus (*B*). Brain MRI axial FLAIR image shows a right frontal parasagittal venous infarct (*arrow, C*). DWI (*arrow, D*) and ADC (*arrow, E*) scans show a right frontal acute venous infarction. Contrast-enhanced T1 sagittal (*F*) and coronal (*G*) images show hypointense flow voids in the superior sagittal sinus and right transverse sinus (*arrows*). MR venography shows absence of venous flow (*arrows*) in the right transverse sinus, sigmoid sinus, right internal jugular vein (*H*, coronal), and superior sagittal sinus (*I*, lateral).

of pregnancy-related cerebral hemorrhage are preeclampsia-eclampsia, followed by arteriovenous malformations and aneurysms.

The risk of aneurysmal rupture increases with gestational age, peaking at 30 to 34 weeks. Cerebral aneurysmal rupture during pregnancy is associated with high maternal (35%) and fetal (17%) mortality.[81] If a ruptured aneurysm is left unsecured surgically, there is a very high rate of recurrent hemorrhage and maternal and fetal mortality, 63% and 27%, respectively. These mortalities were lowered to 11% and 5%, respectively, by early surgery.[81] Thus, if aneurysmal subarachnoid hemorrhage occurs during pregnancy, then surgical control of the aneurysm should be performed immediately during pregnancy, when possible.[82] If urgent obstetric issues prevent immediate neurosurgery, then urgent cesarean delivery is recommended, followed by surgical control of the cerebral aneurysm. There is increased risk of aneurysmal rupture near term. Therefore, it is recommended that unruptured aneurysms at significant risk of rupture be secured before pregnancy, when possible.

Hemorrhage is the most common presenting manifestation of arteriovenous malformations (AVM), followed by seizures or focal neurologic deficits. Whether AVMs bleed more during pregnancy has been debated. A study from 1990 showed an annual rate of hemorrhage of 3.5% in women with AVM and no prior hemorrhage, and 5.8% in those with prior hemorrhage, with no increase secondary to pregnancy.[83] However, when considering the daily risk of rupture, there was a several-fold increase in risk on the day of delivery.[84,85] More recent studies have shown an increase in the rate of intracranial hemorrhage in women during pregnancy and puerperium. A retrospective Chinese study of 264 women with AVM showed an annualized rate of AVM rupture and hemorrhage of 5.59% in pregnant women as compared with 2.52% in nonpregnant women ($P = .002$).[86] Similar results were seen in an American retrospective cohort of 270 women, showing an annual hemorrhage rate of 5.7% in pregnant women versus 1.3% in nonpregnant women (P<.001).[87] Further, AVM bleeding during pregnancy is associated with a higher rebleeding rate than in nonpregnant women (26% vs 6%, respectively).

Regarding management of AVMs in pregnancy, based on the considerations discussed earlier, expert recommendation are that (1) if a woman with known AVM anticipates pregnancy, the AVM should be treated before pregnancy; (2) if an AVM is discovered during pregnancy and has not bled during the pregnancy, then conservative observation is usually recommended with plans to proceed to definitive treatment after delivery; and (3) if an AVM bleeds during pregnancy, then consideration should be given to treatment during the pregnancy, taking into account the grade of the lesion and the expected timing of benefit in lowering risk (immediate for low-grade lesions amenable to complete surgical excision or embolization) but delayed by 1 to 3 years for higher-grade lesions requiring radiosurgery and combination therapies.[88] Cesarean delivery is usually favored over vaginal delivery due to higher rates of hemorrhage on the day of delivery.

MANAGEMENT OF STROKE IN PREGNANCY
Acute Ischemic Stroke Management

For nonpregnant patients with acute ischemic stroke, early thrombolytic therapy and endovascular clot retrieval are the recommended hyperacute therapies to improve long-term clinical outcomes. However, these therapies have not been studied in randomized trials involving pregnant women. Further, this therapy is often withheld in many women, given concerns for life-threatening maternal and placental hemorrhages, including risk of fetal demise. The most widespread used thrombolytic, tissue plasminogen activator, does not cross the placenta and therefore, does not cause direct fetal harm. There have been numerous case reports and small case series of use of thrombolytic therapy for arterial ischemic stroke and other systemic indications, without clear evidence of harm or benefit.[89] A recent study sought to address this question. Using data from the AHA Get with the Guidelines Registry, the investigators compared 338 pregnant or postpartum women with 24,303 women, all acute ischemic stroke sufferers who received reperfusion therapy (intravenous thrombolytic or catheter-based thrombolysis/clot retrieval). Pregnant women were less likely to receive intravenous thrombolysis than the nonpregnant women, but the overall rates of reperfusion therapy were similar between the 2 groups. Furthermore, patients in both groups had similar rates of discharge to home. There was a nonsignificant trend of increased rates of symptomatic intracranial hemorrhage in pregnant women who received intravenous thrombolysis as compared with nonpregnant women. Fetal outcomes were not reported in this study. However, this study did show that it may be reasonable to offer reperfusion to pregnant/postpartum women who suffered an ischemic stroke. Intra-arterial therapy is an especially interesting approach to acute stroke management in this population.[90]

Delivery

The timing of delivery for women who have suffered a stroke during pregnancy is determined by the severity of the mother's medical condition and fetal stability. For women who suffer a stroke at less than 24 weeks' gestation, decisions regarding continuing pregnancy versus therapeutic termination rely on the clinical state of the patient and the need for use of thrombolysis, which can increase the risk of fetal loss. For women who suffer a stroke at 24 to 32 weeks' gestation, antenatal glucocorticoids may be given to accelerate fetal lung maturation. If mother and fetus are clinically stable, then pregnancy may be continued, aiming for controlled induction at 34 to 39 weeks' gestation. Cesarean section should be avoided if possible.[91]

Secondary Stroke Prevention of Ischemic Stroke in Pregnancy/Puerperium

The choice of antithrombotic will be determined by the stroke mechanism and patient preferences. Aspirin is by far the most widely used antithrombotic for secondary stroke prevention. It is deemed safe for use in the second and third trimesters for fetus and mother. In the first trimester, however, aspirin use has been reported to have an association with increased incidence of fetal gastroschisis and other fetal malformations.[92] Other studies and meta-analyses of aspirin use for prevention of preeclampsia even before 11 weeks do not support the same findings. A large meta-analysis of studies of antiplatelet use in women at high risk for preeclampsia showed safety of antiplatelets without adverse fetal outcomes, increase in fetal systemic or intracranial hemorrhages, and adverse effects on fetal weight and with more favorable maternal outcomes.[93] The safety of other antiplatelets during pregnancy has not been established in clinical trials.

Regarding anticoagulants, warfarin is contraindicated in pregnancy due to its teratogenic effects and risk for fetal hemorrhages. It should be avoided in early pregnancy, and if at all also throughout the entire pregnancy because it may also cause central nervous system abnormalities in the second and third trimesters. Preference should be given to heparins. Unfractionated heparin (UFH) and LMWH do not cross the placenta, although UFH can increase the risk of maternal thrombocytopenia and osteoporosis. The novel oral anticoagulants should not be used during pregnancy, given their uncertain safety profile. Postdelivery, nursing mothers may continue to take low-dose aspirin, warfarin, UFH, and LMWH. However, novel oral anticoagulants are not recommended.[92,94]

STROKE OUTCOMES
Morbidity and Mortality

Stroke morbidity is determined by the type of stroke, its severity, and therapies received for early management and secondary prevention. Mortality rates for stroke in pregnancy are reported at 2.7% to 20.4% and have not significantly changed over the past decades, despite advances in stroke treatment.[1]

Risk of Recurrent Stroke

For women of child-bearing age who have a stroke or VST, the risk of a recurrent stroke during pregnancy is not substantially high. A study of 441 women with a first ever stroke followed for 5 years showed that only 13 strokes occurred in that time; only 2 strokes occurred during pregnancy/puerperium. Puerperium was the period of highest risk for an obstetric ischemic stroke. Therefore, having had a previous ischemic stroke should not preclude women of child-bearing age to seek pregnancy.[95] However, women with prior stroke who become pregnant seem to have a significantly higher risk of miscarriages, fetal loss, and pregnancy complications than pregnant women without prior stroke. This study did not determine the cause of this association, although it is postulated that the underlying cause of the index stroke could affect fertility, such as in patients with antiphospholipid syndrome or other hypercoagulable states.[96]

REFERENCES

1. Swartz RH, Cayley ML, Foley N, et al. The incidence of pregnancy-related stroke: a systematic review and meta-analysis. Int J Stroke 2017;12(7):687–97.
2. Kuklina EV, Tong X, Bansil P, et al. Trends in pregnancy hospitalizations that included a stroke in the United States from 1994 to 2007: reasons for concern? Stroke 2011;42(9):2564–70.
3. Ban L, Sprigg N, Abdul Sultan A, et al. Incidence of first stroke in pregnant and nonpregnant women of childbearing age: a population-based cohort study from England. J Am Heart Assoc 2017;6(4) [pii:e004601].
4. Kamel H, Navi BB, Sriram N, et al. Risk of a thrombotic event after the 6-week postpartum period. N Engl J Med 2014;370(14):1307–15.
5. James AH, Bushnell CD, Jamison MG, et al. Incidence and risk factors for stroke in pregnancy and the puerperium. Obstet Gynecol 2005;106(3):509–16.
6. Miller EC, Gatollari HJ, Too G, et al. Risk of pregnancy-associated stroke across age groups in New York state. JAMA Neurol 2016;73(12):1461–7.
7. Qureshi AI, Saeed O, Malik AA, et al. Pregnancy in advanced age and the risk of stroke in postmenopausal women: analysis of Women's Health Initiative Study. Am J Obstet Gynecol 2017;216(4):409.e1-6.
8. Miller EC, Gallo M, Kulick ER, et al. Infections and risk of peripartum stroke during delivery admissions. Stroke 2018;49(5):1129–34.
9. Sanders BD, Davis MG, Holley SL, et al. Pregnancy-associated stroke. J Midwifery Womens Health 2018;63(1):23–32.
10. Dayan N, Filion KB, Okano M, et al. Cardiovascular risk following fertility therapy: systematic review and meta-analysis. J Am Coll Cardiol 2017;70(10):1203–13.
11. Udell JA, Lu H, Redelmeier DA. Failure of fertility therapy and subsequent adverse cardiovascular events. CMAJ 2017;189(10):E391–7.
12. Lanska DJ, Kryscio RJ. Risk factors for peripartum and postpartum stroke and intracranial venous thrombosis. Stroke 2000;31(6):1274–82.
13. Lin SY, Hu CJ, Lin HC. Increased risk of stroke in patients who undergo cesarean section delivery: a nationwide population-based study. Am J Obstet Gynecol 2008;198(4):391.e1-7.
14. Sanghavi M, Rutherford JD. Cardiovascular physiology of pregnancy. Circulation 2014;130(12):1003–8.
15. Feske SK, Singhal AB. Cerebrovascular disorders complicating pregnancy. Continuum (Minneap Minn) 2014;20(1 Neurology of Pregnancy):80–99.
16. Poppas A, Shroff SG, Korcarz CE, et al. Serial assessment of the cardiovascular system in normal pregnancy. Role of arterial compliance and pulsatile arterial load. Circulation 1997;95(10):2407–15.
17. Brenner B. Haemostatic changes in pregnancy. Thromb Res 2004;114(5–6): 409–14.
18. Coutinho T, Lamai O, Nerenberg K. Hypertensive disorders of pregnancy and cardiovascular diseases: current knowledge and future directions. Curr Treat Options Cardiovasc Med 2018;20(7):56.
19. Ray JG, Vermeulen MJ, Schull MJ, et al. Cardiovascular health after maternal placental syndromes (CHAMPS): population-based retrospective cohort study. Lancet 2005;366(9499):1797–803.
20. Wu P, Haththotuwa R, Kwok CS, et al. Preeclampsia and future cardiovascular health: a systematic review and meta-analysis. Circ Cardiovasc Qual Outcomes 2017;10(2) [pii:e003497].

21. Umesawa M, Kobashi G. Epidemiology of hypertensive disorders in pregnancy: prevalence, risk factors, predictors and prognosis. Hypertens Res 2017;40(3): 213–20.
22. Kuklina EV, Ayala C, Callaghan WM. Hypertensive disorders and severe obstetric morbidity in the United States. Obstet Gynecol 2009;113(6):1299–306.
23. Miller EC, Gatollari HJ, Too G, et al. Risk factors for pregnancy-associated stroke in women with preeclampsia. Stroke 2017;48(7):1752–9.
24. Steegers EA, von Dadelszen P, Duvekot JJ, et al. Pre-eclampsia. Lancet 2010; 376(9741):631–44.
25. Bateman BT, Schumacher HC, Bushnell CD, et al. Intracerebral hemorrhage in pregnancy: frequency, risk factors, and outcome. Neurology 2006;67(3):424–9.
26. Leffert LR, Clancy CR, Bateman BT, et al. Hypertensive disorders and pregnancy-related stroke: frequency, trends, risk factors, and outcomes. Obstet Gynecol 2015;125(1):124–31.
27. Brown MA, Magee LA, Kenny LC, et al. Hypertensive disorders of pregnancy: ISSHP classification, diagnosis, and management recommendations for international practice. Hypertension 2018;72(1):24–43.
28. Bushnell C, Chireau M. Preeclampsia and stroke: risks during and after pregnancy. Stroke Res Treat 2011;2011:858134.
29. Rodie VA, Freeman DJ, Sattar N, et al. Pre-eclampsia and cardiovascular disease: metabolic syndrome of pregnancy? Atherosclerosis 2004;175(2):189–202.
30. MacKay AP, Berg CJ, Atrash HK. Pregnancy-related mortality from preeclampsia and eclampsia. Obstet Gynecol 2001;97(4):533–8.
31. Bellamy L, Casas JP, Hingorani AD, et al. Pre-eclampsia and risk of cardiovascular disease and cancer in later life: systematic review and meta-analysis. BMJ 2007;335(7627):974.
32. Crandon AJ, Isherwood DM. Effect of aspirin on incidence of pre-eclampsia. Lancet 1979;1(8130):1356.
33. Rolnik DL, Wright D, Poon LC, et al. Aspirin versus placebo in pregnancies at high risk for preterm preeclampsia. N Engl J Med 2017;377(7):613–22.
34. Hofmeyr GJ, Lawrie TA, Atallah AN, et al. Calcium supplementation during pregnancy for preventing hypertensive disorders and related problems. Cochrane Database Syst Rev 2014;(6):CD001059.
35. Bassaw B, Roopnarinesingh S, Roopnarinesingh A, et al. Prevention of hypertensive disorders of pregnancy. J Obstet Gynaecol 1998;18(2):123–6.
36. Villar J, Repke JT. Calcium supplementation during pregnancy may reduce preterm delivery in high-risk populations. Am J Obstet Gynecol 1990;163(4 Pt 1): 1124–31.
37. American College of Obstetricians and Gynecologists, Task Force on Hypertension in Pregnancy. Hypertension in pregnancy. Report of the American College of Obstetricians and Gynecologists' Task Force on Hypertension in Pregnancy. Obstet Gynecol 2013;122(5):1122–31.
38. Bushnell C, McCullough LD, Awad IA, et al. Guidelines for the prevention of stroke in women: a statement for healthcare professionals from the American Heart Association/American Stroke Association. Stroke 2014;45(5):1545–88.
39. Magee LA, von Dadelszen P, Rey E, et al. Less-tight versus tight control of hypertension in pregnancy. N Engl J Med 2015;372(5):407–17.
40. Altman D, Carroli G, Duley L, et al. Do women with pre-eclampsia, and their babies, benefit from magnesium sulphate? The Magpie Trial: a randomised placebo-controlled trial. Lancet 2002;359(9321):1877–90.

41. Which anticonvulsant for women with eclampsia? Evidence from the Collaborative Eclampsia Trial. Lancet 1995;345(8963):1455–63.
42. Lucas MJ, Leveno KJ, Cunningham FG. A comparison of magnesium sulfate with phenytoin for the prevention of eclampsia. N Engl J Med 1995;333(4):201–5.
43. McDermott M, Miller EC, Rundek T, et al. Preeclampsia: association with posterior reversible encephalopathy syndrome and stroke. Stroke 2018;49(3):524–30.
44. Brewer J, Owens MY, Wallace K, et al. Posterior reversible encephalopathy syndrome in 46 of 47 patients with eclampsia. Am J Obstet Gynecol 2013;208(6):468.e1-6.
45. Mayama M, Uno K, Tano S, et al. Incidence of posterior reversible encephalopathy syndrome in eclamptic and patients with preeclampsia with neurologic symptoms. Am J Obstet Gynecol 2016;215(2):239.e1-5.
46. Bartynski WS, Boardman JF. Distinct imaging patterns and lesion distribution in posterior reversible encephalopathy syndrome. AJNR Am J Neuroradiol 2007;28(7):1320–7.
47. Liman TG, Bohner G, Heuschmann PU, et al. Clinical and radiological differences in posterior reversible encephalopathy syndrome between patients with preeclampsia-eclampsia and other predisposing diseases. Eur J Neurol 2012;19(7):935–43.
48. Postma IR, Slager S, Kremer HP, et al. Long-term consequences of the posterior reversible encephalopathy syndrome in eclampsia and preeclampsia: a review of the obstetric and nonobstetric literature. Obstet Gynecol Surv 2014;69(5):287–300.
49. Call GK, Fleming MC, Sealfon S, et al. Reversible cerebral segmental vasoconstriction. Stroke 1988;19(9):1159–70.
50. Calabrese LH, Dodick DW, Schwedt TJ, et al. Narrative review: reversible cerebral vasoconstriction syndromes. Ann Intern Med 2007;146(1):34–44.
51. Ducros A, Boukobza M, Porcher R, et al. The clinical and radiological spectrum of reversible cerebral vasoconstriction syndrome. A prospective series of 67 patients. Brain 2007;130(Pt 12):3091–101.
52. Singhal AB. Cerebral vasoconstriction syndromes. Top Stroke Rehabil 2004;11(2):1–6.
53. Singhal AB, Hajj-Ali RA, Topcuoglu MA, et al. Reversible cerebral vasoconstriction syndromes: analysis of 139 cases. Arch Neurol 2011;68(8):1005–12.
54. Singhal AB, Topcuoglu MA, Fok JW, et al. RCVS and PACNS: Clinical, imaging, and angiographic comparison. Ann Neurol 2016;79(6):882–94.
55. Chen SP, Fuh JL, Lirng JF, et al. Recurrent primary thunderclap headache and benign CNS angiopathy: spectra of the same disorder? Neurology 2006;67(12):2164–9.
56. Ducros A. Reversible cerebral vasoconstriction syndrome. Lancet Neurol 2012;11(10):906–17.
57. Singhal AB. Postpartum angiopathy with reversible posterior leukoencephalopathy. Arch Neurol 2004;61(3):411–6.
58. Singhal AB, Caviness VS, Begleiter AF, et al. Cerebral vasoconstriction and stroke after use of serotonergic drugs. Neurology 2002;58(1):130–3.
59. Nighoghossian N, Derex L, Trouillas P. Multiple intracerebral hemorrhages and vasospasm following antimigrainous drug abuse. Headache 1998;38(6):478–80.
60. Razavi M, Bendixen B, Maley JE, et al. CNS pseudovasculitis in a patient with pheochromocytoma. Neurology 1999;52(5):1088–90.
61. Verillaud B, Ducros A, Massiou H, et al. Reversible cerebral vasoconstriction syndrome in two patients with a carotid glomus tumour. Cephalalgia 2010;30(10):1271–5.

62. Fugate JE, Wijdicks EF, Parisi JE, et al. Fulminant postpartum cerebral vasoconstriction syndrome. Arch Neurol 2012;69(1):111–7.

63. Lee JH, Martin NA, Alsina G, et al. Hemodynamically significant cerebral vasospasm and outcome after head injury: a prospective study. J Neurosurg 1997; 87(2):221–33.

64. Wolff V, Lauer V, Rouyer O, et al. Cannabis use, ischemic stroke, and multifocal intracranial vasoconstriction: a prospective study in 48 consecutive young patients. Stroke 2011;42(6):1778–80.

65. Ducros A, Fiedler U, Porcher R, et al. Hemorrhagic manifestations of reversible cerebral vasoconstriction syndrome: frequency, features, and risk factors. Stroke 2010;41(11):2505–11.

66. Dodick DW. Reversible segmental cerebral vasoconstriction (Call-Fleming syndrome): the role of calcium antagonists. Cephalalgia 2003;23(3):163–5.

67. Kumar S, Goddeau RP Jr, Selim MH, et al. Atraumatic convexal subarachnoid hemorrhage: clinical presentation, imaging patterns, and etiologies. Neurology 2010;74(11):893–9.

68. Chen SP, Fuh JL, Wang SJ, et al. Magnetic resonance angiography in reversible cerebral vasoconstriction syndromes. Ann Neurol 2010;67(5):648–56.

69. Hajj-Ali RA, Furlan A, Abou-Chebel A, et al. Benign angiopathy of the central nervous system: cohort of 16 patients with clinical course and long-term followup. Arthritis Rheum 2002;47(6):662–9.

70. Singhal AB, Kimberly WT, Schaefer PW, et al. Case records of the Massachusetts General Hospital. Case 8-2009. A 36-year-old woman with headache, hypertension, and seizure 2 weeks post partum. N Engl J Med 2009;360(11):1126–37.

71. Bousser MG, Ferro JM. Cerebral venous thrombosis: an update. Lancet Neurol 2007;6(2):162–70.

72. Ferro JM, Canhao P, Stam J, et al. Prognosis of cerebral vein and dural sinus thrombosis: results of the International Study on Cerebral Vein and Dural Sinus Thrombosis (ISCVT). Stroke 2004;35(3):664–70.

73. Biousse V, Ameri A, Bousser MG. Isolated intracranial hypertension as the only sign of cerebral venous thrombosis. Neurology 1999;53(7):1537–42.

74. Ferro JM, Correia M, Pontes C, et al. Cerebral vein and dural sinus thrombosis in Portugal: 1980-1998. Cerebrovasc Dis 2001;11(3):177–82.

75. Cumurciuc R, Crassard I, Sarov M, et al. Headache as the only neurological sign of cerebral venous thrombosis: a series of 17 cases. J Neurol Neurosurg Psychiatry 2005;76(8):1084–7.

76. Idbaih A, Boukobza M, Crassard I, et al. MRI of clot in cerebral venous thrombosis: high diagnostic value of susceptibility-weighted images. Stroke 2006;37(4):991–5.

77. Yuh WT, Simonson TM, Wang AM, et al. Venous sinus occlusive disease: MR findings. AJNR Am J Neuroradiol 1994;15(2):309–16.

78. Canhao P, Ferro JM, Lindgren AG, et al. Causes and predictors of death in cerebral venous thrombosis. Stroke 2005;36(8):1720–5.

79. Aguiar de Sousa D, Canhao P, Crassard I, et al. Safety of pregnancy after cerebral venous thrombosis: results of the ISCVT (International Study on Cerebral Vein and Dural Sinus Thrombosis)-2 PREGNANCY Study. Stroke 2017;48(11):3130–3.

80. Kittner SJ, Stern BJ, Feeser BR, et al. Pregnancy and the risk of stroke. N Engl J Med 1996;335:768–74.

81. Dias MS, Sekhar LN. Intracranial hemorrhage from aneurysms and arteriovenous malformations during pregnancy and the puerperium. Neurosurgery 1990;27: 855–65.

82. Meyers PM, Halbach VV, Malek AM, et al. Endovascular treatment of cerebral artery aneurysms during pregnancy: report of three cases. AJNR Am J Neuroradiol 2000;21:1306–11.

83. Horton JC, Chambers WA, Lyons SL, et al. Pregnancy and the risk of hemorrhage from cerebral arteriovenous malformations. Neurosurgery 1990;27:867–72.

84. Parkinson D, Bachers G. Arteriovenous malformations: summary of 100 consecutive supratentorial cases. J Neurosurg 1980;53:285–99.

85. Weir B, Macdonald L. Management of intracranial aneurysms and arteriovenous malformations during pregnancy. In: Wilkins RH, Rengachary SS, editors. Neurosurgery. New York: McGraw-Hill; 1996. p. 2421–7.

86. Zhu D, Zhao P, Lv N, et al. Rupture risk of cerebral arteriovenous malformations during pregnancy and puerperium: a single-center experience and pooled data analysis. World Neurosurg 2018;111:e308–15.

87. Porras JL, Yang W, Philadelphia E, et al. Hemorrhage risk of brain arteriovenous malformations during pregnancy and puerperium in a North American Cohort. Stroke 2017;48(6):1507–13.

88. Ogilvy CS, Stieg PE, Awad I, et al. Recommendations for the management of intracranial arteriovenous malformations: a statement for healthcare professionals for a special writing group of the Stroke Council, American Stroke Association. Stroke 2001;32:1458–71.

89. Shainker SA, Edlow JA, O'Brien K. Cerebrovascular emergencies in pregnancy. Best Pract Res Clin Obstet Gynaecol 2015;29(5):721–31.

90. Leffert LR, Clancy CR, Bateman BT, et al. Treatment patterns and short-term outcomes in ischemic stroke in pregnancy or postpartum period. Am J Obstet Gynecol 2016;214(6):723.e1-11.

91. Lee M-J, Hickenbottom S. Cerebrovascular disorders complicating pregnancy. In: Biller JL, Lockwood CJ, editors. UpToDate. Waltham (MA): UpToDate; 2018.

92. Caso V, Falorni A, Bushnell CD, et al. Pregnancy, hormonal treatments for infertility, contraception, and menopause in women after ischemic stroke: a consensus document. Stroke 2017;48(2):501–6.

93. Duley L, Henderson-Smart D, Knight M, et al. Antiplatelet drugs for prevention of pre-eclampsia and its consequences: systematic review. BMJ 2001;322(7282): 329–33.

94. Bates SM, Greer IA, Middeldorp S, et al. VTE, thrombophilia, antithrombotic therapy, and pregnancy: antithrombotic therapy and prevention of thrombosis, 9th ed: American College of Chest Physicians Evidence-Based Clinical Practice Guidelines. Chest 2012;141(2 Suppl):e691S–736S.

95. Lamy C, Hamon JB, Coste J, et al. Ischemic stroke in young women: risk of recurrence during subsequent pregnancies. French Study Group on Stroke in Pregnancy. Neurology 2000;55(2):269–74.

96. van Alebeek ME, de Vrijer M, Arntz RM, et al. Increased risk of pregnancy complications after stroke: the FUTURE study (follow-up of transient ischemic attack and stroke patients and unelucidated risk factor evaluation). Stroke 2018;49(4): 877–83.

Moving?

Make sure your subscription moves with you!

To notify us of your new address, find your **Clinics Account Number** (located on your mailing label above your name), and contact customer service at:

Email: journalscustomerservice-usa@elsevier.com

800-654-2452 (subscribers in the U.S. & Canada)
314-447-8871 (subscribers outside of the U.S. & Canada)

Fax number: 314-447-8029

Elsevier Health Sciences Division
Subscription Customer Service
3251 Riverport Lane
Maryland Heights, MO 63043

*To ensure uninterrupted delivery of your subscription, please notify us at least 4 weeks in advance of move.

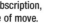

Moving?

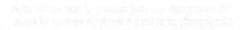

Printed and bound by CPI Group (UK) Ltd, Croydon, CR0 4YY

07/10/2024

01040501-0014